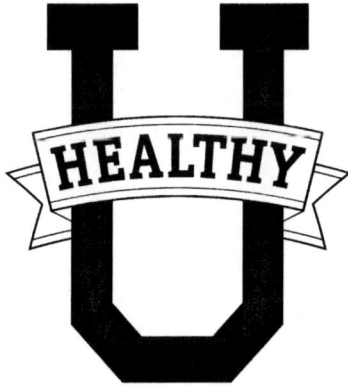

HEALTHY U

A quick reference guide to eating healthy on campus and beating the Freshman 15

Melanie M. Jatsek, RD, LD

Good For You Press
Cleveland, OH

Healthy U
*A quick reference guide to eating healthy on campus
and beating the Freshman 15*

© 2011 Melanie M. Jatsek

Published by
Good For You Press

To order additional copies go to:

www.healthyUbook.com

Cover and interior design by
Peri Poloni-Gabriel, Knockout Design, www.knockoutbooks.com

ISBN-13: 978-0-9833941-0-5
LCCN: 2011923620

First Edition
Printed in the United States of America

CONTENTS

APPENDIX: *continued*

INTRODUCTION

Seventy percent of college students gain about 9 pounds during their first and second years (2005 study by the Journal of American College Health). Eighty-five percent report feeling stressed on a daily basis, while six out of 10 report having felt so stressed they couldn't get their work done on one or more occasions (Poll conducted by the Associated Press and MTV-U). Could this happen to you? Is this happening to you right now? *Healthy U* will help you beat it.

As a college student living in my own apartment for the first time, I made lots of poor choices. With the exception of walking to and from classes, exercise was pretty much nonexistent. My kitchen cabinets were loaded with packaged snacks like cream-filled snack cakes. I ate sugar-coated cereal for breakfast, pancakes with syrup for dinner and snacked on white bread and potato chips in between. It's no wonder I struggled to stay awake in classes and was sick all the time! I wrote this book because I wish I'd had one like it when I was in college. If I knew then what I know now, things would have been a lot easier for me. That's what this book will do for you—make your life easier. *Healthy U* will show you how to make food work for you rather than against you. This way of eating will help you to:

✔ Fit into your shorts and swimsuit at spring break

✔ Get a better night's sleep

✔ Avoid getting colds, the flu and other common illnesses

✓ Score better on exams

✓ Have more energy and be more productive

✓ Feel more emotionally balanced and less stressed out

✓ And, ultimately, get through college without packing on extra pounds

Whether you're a first-year or fourth-year student, don't wait until you're walking across the stage on graduation day to start making healthier choices. Start now. Start today. Don't join the thirty-four percent of people in this country who are obese and suffering the many health consequences that go hand in hand with being overweight. Your college years can be some of the best years of your life. By learning just a few simple secrets about eating right, you can have more fun and get better grades, too.

Healthy U includes 21 "Secrets" to help make college life easier. Relying on the most current nutrition recommendations, each Secret shows you simple steps you can take to make better food choices and form healthier eating habits. You'll also find helpful nutrition tips, easy-to-read nutrition facts, meal ideas, foods to beware of and foods to eat more of, all while answering the "what's in it for me?" question. At the conclusion of each Secret, you're encouraged to put what you learned into action by building Power Habits™. Pick whichever ones (or just one) you're most comfortable with and record it on the Power Habit™ Tracking Chart in the back of the book. Over time, the more Power Habits™ you build, the more prepared you'll be to jump over any hurdle that stands in your way.

Secret 1:

READ IT BEFORE YOU EAT IT!

What's in it for you?

✓ Learn how to make healthier food choices instantly

✓ Fit into your skinny jeans . . . without having to lie on the floor to zip them up

Fast food, late nights, caffeine, cramming for tests and more home-work than you knew was possible are typical challenges for most college students. It's no wonder you're *stressed out*! One of the secrets to handling this stress and having more energy is learning how to make better choices about what you eat and drink.

The best place to start is the food label. Choosing healthier foods will be a breeze when you understand how to read the label.

*Eating healthy isn't an all-or-nothing game. ...
In the end, it's about balance*

Macronutrients and micronutrients

Macronutrients

There are three nutrients in food that supply energy (calories): fat, carbohydrate and protein. Some foods, like 2% milk, are a combination of all three, while others, like an apple, primarily contain only one macronutrient in this case, carbohydrates.

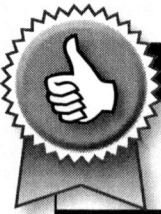

> **GOOD IDEA!**
>
> *To feel full for a little longer, toss a small handful of walnuts into your morning bowl of oatmeal!*

1. **Fat**

   Supplying 9 calories per gram, dietary fat is the most concentrated source of energy. (You'll learn in Secret 2: Get Smart, Eat Fat that certain fats, such as polyunsaturated and monounsaturated, are better for you than others.) Although many people think they should eat a fat-free diet, this is a myth. Fat carries out several important functions in your body, including:

   ✓ Dissolving key fat-soluble vitamins (Vitamins A, D, E and K) so that your body can use them

   ✓ Helping you feel full after eating

   ✓ Protecting your organs

   ✓ Insulating your body

   Monounsaturated and polyunsaturated fats are found in oils, nuts, seeds, nut butters, avocados and olives. These are considered "good" fats. The "bad" fats are saturated fat and trans fat. By reading labels, you can avoid these fats that are known to raise your cholesterol levels and increase your chances of developing heart disease or having a stroke.

   Cholesterol is a waxy substance found only in animal products. While it's gotten a bad reputation, it actually performs some important functions in your body, like forming cell membranes and hormones. Fortunately, your body makes all the cholesterol it needs. That means you don't need to eat anything that contains cholesterol. Ironically, studies have shown that dietary cholesterol doesn't have a strong impact on raising blood cholesterol levels, but eating saturated and trans fats can contribute to unhealthy cholesterol levels and are known to cause other health problems. The American Heart Association recommends keeping your dietary cholesterol below 300 milligrams (mg) per day.

2. *Carbohydrate*

Carbohydrates have 4 calories per gram. They supply your entire body (most notably your brain) with the energy you need to go about your day and for physical activities like dancing, swimming, running and climbing the stairs when the elevator isn't working. Carbohydrates are in fruits, vegetables, milk, yogurt, grains, beans and legumes.

On the food label, you'll notice that fiber and sugars are listed under total carbohydrate. These are two of the three types of carbohydrates. The third is starches. Although your body can't digest fiber, it's still an important part of a healthy diet. Have you ever experienced a lasting full feeling after eating a bowl of Frosted Mini-Wheats? If so, you can thank fiber. Fiber helps to keep you full longer because it stays in your stomach longer. Insoluble fiber, also known as "roughage", helps to prevent constipation because it keeps the digestion process in your intestines moving. Whole-wheat products, wheat bran, vegetables, legumes and fruit skins all contain insoluble fiber. Meanwhile, soluble fiber helps to lower your blood cholesterol levels. To get more soluble fiber, eat oats, legumes, barley, apples, citrus fruits, strawberries and carrots. Most Americans get only from 10 to 15 grams of fiber a day, but you should aim for 25 to 35 grams if you want the health benefits.

Sugars are simple carbohydrates. They occur naturally in foods such as fresh fruit and 100% fruit juices or in the form of refined sugars like corn syrup and white table sugar. Most of the sugars in the American diet are refined. In fact, according to the 2001–04 National Health and Nutrition Examination Survey (NHANES), Americans are averaging about 22.2 teaspoons of sugar a day! That's the amount of sugar in two cans of soda.

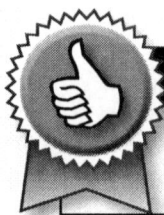

GOOD IDEA!

Buy several varieties of canned beans, like black, pinto and kidney beans. Rinse them under cold water and add to salads or soups to boost your fiber.

3. Protein

With 4 calories per gram, protein helps build your muscles, blood, nails, skin, hair and organs. It's found in dairy products, meat and poultry, fish, soy products, eggs, nuts, seeds, beans and legumes. Chances are you don't need as much protein as you think. The daily guidelines for adults are as follows:

✓ For inactive adults, 0.4 grams of protein per pound of body weight

✓ For recreational exercisers, 0.5-0.7 grams of protein per pound of body weight

✓ For endurance athletes, 0.6-0.7 grams of protein per pound of body weight

✓ For adults building muscle mass, 0.7-0.8 grams of protein per pound of body weight

Micronutrients

These nutrients consist of vitamins and minerals. Although they don't supply calories, your body depends on them to stay healthy and strong.

1. Sodium

Sodium is overabundant in the average American's diet. You need some, but probably much less than you're eating on a daily basis. Sodium is important for maintaining fluid balance, regulating blood pressure, helping muscles relax and transmitting nerve impulses. But too much can contribute to high blood pressure, which can lead to heart disease and stroke.

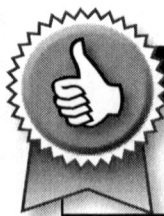

GOOD IDEA!

Use fresh herbs and unsalted spices to season your food without adding sodium.

You probably don't think those salty potato chips you're snacking on have the potential to lead to bone loss over time, but studies have shown that too much sodium can cause you to lose calcium in your urine, which can eventually increase your risk for bone fractures. The American Heart Association recommends keeping your sodium below 2,300 mg a day. That's about 1 teaspoon of salt. The majority of packaged foods contain some sodium so it's easy to exceed the daily recommendation unless you are vigilantly reading labels and selecting food with no or low sodium.

2. *Potassium*

Abundant in fruits, vegetables, milk, fresh meat, poultry and fish, potassium helps regulate fluid balance and blood pressure, transmits nerve impulses and helps your muscles contract. The fewer processed foods you eat, the higher your potassium intake will be.

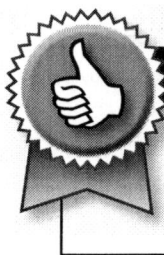

GOOD IDEA!

For a healthy dose of potassium, calcium and the antioxidants vitamin A and C, the next time you order a smoothie ask for skim milk, carrots, oranges and strawberries.

3. *Vitamin A*

Found in both plants and animals, vitamin A helps you see in the dark, promotes cell and tissue health and protects you from infection. When it comes from plants (in the form of carotenoids), it's a powerful antioxidant, offering protection against certain cancers and other diseases. Animal sources of vitamin A (in the form of retinol) include liver, fish oil, eggs, milk fortified with vitamin A and other fortified foods. In plants, you'll find it in yellow, orange and red vegetables and dark leafy greens.

4. *Vitamin C*

Also an antioxidant, vitamin C forms connective tissue, fights infection and keeps your gums and capillaries healthy. It also helps your body do a better job of absorbing the iron from the foods you eat. Vitamin C is in citrus fruits, bell peppers, broccoli, strawberries, cantaloupe, potatoes and tomatoes.

**Sample label for
Macaroni & Cheese**

Nutrition Facts

Serving Size 1 cup (228 g)

Servings Per Container 2

Amount Per Serving

Calories 250	**Calories from Fat** 110

	% Daily Value*
Total Fat 12g	**18%**
Saturated Fat 3g	**15%**
Trans Fat 3 g	
Cholesterol 30mg	**10%**
Sodium 470mg	**20%**
Total Carbohydrate 31g	**10%**
Dietary Fiber 0g	**0%**
Sugars 5g	
Protein 5g	

Vitamin A	**4%**
Vitamin C	**2%**
Calcium	**20%**
Iron	**4%**

*Percent Daily Values are based on a 2,000 calorie diet. Your Daily Values may be higher or lower depending on your calorie needs.

	Calories:	2,000	2,500
Total Fat	Less than	65g	80g
Saturated Fat	Less than	20g	25g
Cholesterol	Less than	300mg	300mg
Sodium	Less than	2400mg	2400mg
Total Carbohydrate		300g	375g
Dietary Fiber		25g	30g

5. **Calcium**

   Calcium helps your heart to beat, builds and strengthens your bones and teeth, helps your muscles to contract and helps your blood to clot (in a good way). Milk, yogurt, cheese, dark leafy greens, fish with bones, calcium-set tofu and calcium-fortified juices and soy milk are all good sources of calcium.

6. **Iron**

   Iron carries oxygen in your blood and delivers it to every cell in your body. Not getting enough iron can lead to anemia, fatigue and infection. There are two forms of iron in the diet—heme and nonheme. Heme iron is found in meat, fish and poultry, while nonheme iron is found in eggs, grains, nuts, nut butters, seeds, beans, soy products, vegetables and fruits. Keep in mind that your body absorbs heme iron more readily.

7. **Other vitamins and minerals**

   Some foods, like fortified breakfast cereals, have a list of other key vitamins and minerals on their labels. For example, if you pick up a box of Total Raisin Bran, in addition to the above nutrients, you'll find vitamin D, vitamin E, thiamin, riboflavin, niacin, vitamin B6, folic acid, vitamin B12, pantothenic acid, phosphorus, magnesium and zinc. If you don't see this extensive list on a food label, it means that the product contains negligible amounts of these nutrients.

Serving size

The calories and nutrition information on a food label are for the serving size listed at the top. All too often, we eat an entire package not realizing we just ate three or four servings. In the sample label of macaroni and cheese, the calories, fat, cholesterol, sodium, carbohydrate, protein, vitamins and minerals are for 1 cup of macaroni and cheese, not the entire package.

Servings per container

This tells you how many servings the package contains. That package of mac-n-cheese contains two servings, so if you polish off the whole box, you'll be downing 500 calories rather than just the 250 listed for a single serving.

? DID YOU KNOW?

Many packaged foods contain more than one serving per container? This means that if you eat the entire package, you're eating double, triple or even quadruple the calories on the food label. Yikes!

As a freshman, I got into the habit of eating one of those huge prepackaged oatmeal cookies between classes every day. It wasn't until I noticed my jeans getting a little tight that I realized the nutrition facts on the label were for a quarter of the cookie—I was eating four servings!!

—BECKI, senior at Auburn University

Calories and calories from fat

This tells you how many calories are in the food you're about to eat and how many of those calories come from fat. Almost half the calories in the box of mac-n-cheese come from fat.

% Daily Value (% DV)

This shows you how the food fits into a 2,000-calorie diet. Your calorie needs may be more or less than 2,000 and depend on your age, height, weight, activity level and gender. You can calculate it by using any of the online calorie calculators, like the one offered by the Mayo Clinic. You can find it at www.mayoclinic.com/health/calorie-calculator/nu00598. Here's how to approach the numbers:

✓ 5% or less of the Daily Value is low. Aim low when it comes to total fat, saturated fat, cholesterol and sodium.

✓ 20% or more of the Daily Value is high. Aim high when it comes to fiber, vitamins and minerals.

Looking at the % DV, you'll notice that macaroni and cheese is high in sodium and calcium and low in fiber, vitamin A, vitamin C and iron.

All food labels with more than one ingredient have a table explaining the Percent Daily Values for both a 2,000- and 2,500-calorie diet. Here you'll find the recommendations for total fat, saturated fat, cholesterol, sodium, total carbohydrate and fiber. The total fat recommendation for a 2,000-calorie diet is less than 65 grams. Eating one serving of macaroni and cheese (12 grams of fat per serving) means using up 18% of your fat grams for the day.

$$\frac{\textbf{12 grams}}{\textbf{65 grams}} = \textbf{0.18}$$

Overall, macaroni and cheese isn't your best choice for lunch. Eating foods with lots of fat and sodium will make you feel sluggish. Sure, they taste good, but there are plenty of tasty convenient foods that won't put you to sleep. (You'll learn more about these foods in the upcoming Secrets.) Do you have to swear off mac-n-cheese forever? Of course not, but if you want to eat something that will help you concentrate and give you energy, have a salad topped with grilled chicken and a whole grain roll on the side instead.

Trans fat, sugar and protein have no assigned % DV. So choose foods with 0 grams of trans fat and the least amount of sugar (more on why later). Sugar includes both natural sugars (like those found in fruit and milk) and added sugars. Although unsweetened applesauce has 8 grams of sugar per serving, it's a perfectly healthy choice. Unlike the sugar in a can of soda, fruit sugar is natural.

Added sugars can hide out in the ingredients panel in any of these forms:

✧ Brown sugar	✧ High fructose corn syrup	✧ Malt syrup
✧ Corn sweetener	✧ Honey	✧ Maltose
✧ Corn syrup	✧ Sugar	✧ Molasses
✧ Dextrose	✧ Fructose	✧ Raw sugar
✧ Fruit juice concentrates	✧ Invert sugarLactose	✧ Sucrose
✧ Glucose		✧ Syrup

The ingredients list

Ingredients in the largest amounts are listed first. On the sample label of energy drink below, carbonated water is the major ingredient, followed by sucrose and glucose (both sugars). So in other words, when you gulp down a can of your favorite energy drink, what you're really drinking is carbonated sugar water!

Ingredients list of a typical energy drink

Ingredients:

CARBONATED WATER, SUCROSE, GLUCOSE, SODIUM CITRATE
TAURINE, GLUCURONOLACTONE, CAFFEINE, INSTOL,
NIACINAMIDE, CALCIUM PANTOTHENATE, PYRIDOXINE HCL,
VITAMIN B12, ARTIFICIAL FLAVORS, COLORS

Label claims

What does it really mean when a can of soup says "low sodium" or "reduced sodium"? The Food and Drug Administration (FDA) imposes strict guidelines on how certain food-label claims may be used. Here's a list to help you sort through the label lingo:

The Claims

✧ **Low calorie**- less than 40 calories per serving

✧ **Low cholesterol**- less than 20 mg of cholesterol

✧ **Reduced**- 25% less of the specified nutrient or calories than the usual product

✧ **Good source of**- provides at least 10% of the Daily Value of a particular vitamin or nutrient per serving

✧ **Calorie free**- less than 5 calories per serving

✧ **Fat free/sugar free**- less than ½ gram of fat or sugar per serving

✧ **Low sodium**- less than 140 mg of sodium per serving

✧ **High in**- provides 20% or more of the Daily Value of a specified nutrient per serving

✧ **High fiber**- 5 or more grams of fiber per serving

Calculating percentage of calories from carbohydrates, protein and fat

Most foods contain a combination of carbohydrate, protein and fat. Here's a simple three-step calculation to show how much of each is in your favorite foods.

1. ***First you need to know how many calories are in one gram:***

    1 gram of carbohydrate = 4 calories
    1 gram of protein = 4 calories
    1 gram of fat = 9 calories

2. ***To convert grams into calories, multiply the grams of carbohydrate, protein and fat listed on the label by the above numbers. In the macaroni-and-cheese example:***

    31 grams of carbohydrates x 4 = 124 calories
    5 grams of protein x 4 = 20 calories
    12 grams of fat x 9 = 108 calories

3. ***To calculate the percentage, divide the answers from step 2 by the total calories per serving and multiply by 100:***

    124/250 = 0.496 x 100 = 49.6% carbohydrate
    20/250 = 0.08 x 100 = 8% protein
    108/250 = 0.432 x 100 = 43.2% fat

Now take it one step further. The American Heart Association recommends that less than 7% of total calories come from saturated fat. To calculate the percentage of saturated fat in a product, multiply grams of saturated fat by 9, divide by the total calories per serving and multiply by 100. In the macaroni-and-cheese example:

3 grams saturated fat x 9 = 27 calories
27/250 = 0.108 x 100 = 10.8%

Eating mac-n-cheese every day won't make your heart very happy, and it won't keep your body in shape, either.

What do these percentages mean?

A balanced diet should have the optimal blend of carbohydrates, protein and fat. Aim for:

50%-65%   Carbohydrate
15%-30%   Protein
20%-35%   Fat
<7%   Saturated fat

So, how does that package of mac-n-cheese measure up? It's high in total fat (43%) and saturated fat (10.8%), moderate in carbohydrate (49.6%) and low in protein (8%).

READ IT POWER HABITS™!

✓ Read the food labels of every food you consider eating today.

✓ Choose those with a 20% or higher DV for fiber, calcium, iron, vitamin A and/or vitamin C.

✓ Choose those with less than a 20% DV for total fat, saturated fat, cholesterol and/or sodium.

✓ For fun, calculate the percentage of carbohydrate, protein, fat and saturated fat in a couple of food products to see how they match up with the recommendations.

✓ Opt for foods labeled with "Reduced," "Good source of," "High in" and "High fiber".

✓ Write your own Read It Power Habit™: _____

_____

_____

The Bottom Line:

One of the easiest ways to feel good and look great is to make informed decisions instead of picking your foods blindly. Choose the Read It Power Habits™ you're most comfortable with from the list above and put them into action today. Don't forget to record it on your Power Habit™ Tracking Chart in the back of the book!

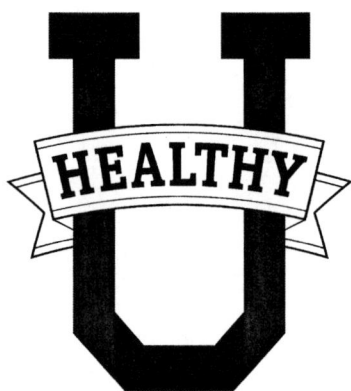

Secret 2:

GET SMART, EAT FAT

What's in it for you?

✓ Learn which fats hijack your brain and how to avoid them

✓ Improve your memory

✓ Learn which fats can make you feel happier

✓ Invest in your future by lowering your risk of heart disease now

Recommendations:

✓ 2 servings (3.5 ounces each) of fatty fish like salmon or light tuna per week

✓ Get less than 7% of your calories from saturated fat (16 grams per 2,000 calories)

✓ Get less than 1% of your calories from trans fat (2 grams per 2,000 calories)

You have a fat head...really!

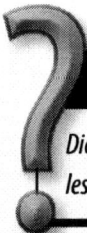

DID YOU KNOW?

Dietary fat won't make you fat unless you eat too much of it. It actually helps you eat less because it keeps you satisfied and makes you feel full.

You have a fat head. Really. Because your brain is two-thirds fat, you need to eat enough fat to give it what it needs. As mentioned earlier, not all fats are created equal. Your brain and your body like some fats better than others. Because fat is so energy-dense, it takes longer to digest. At nine calories per gram (compared with 4 calories per gram for carbohydrates and protein), a little fat goes a long way.

That's why you stay full for hours after eating a cheeseburger and fries but feel like ordering a pizza less than an hour after eating a garden salad. That said, a meal rich in fat makes your body work very hard to digest it. Your heart has to pump more blood to your stomach and intestines, and you have to use more digestive enzymes, which take a lot of energy to create. Ever wonder why you feel like taking a nap after chowing down on four slices of pepperoni pizza? Blame the fat!

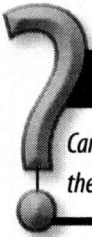

DID YOU KNOW?

Canola oil is made from tiny canola seeds produced by yellow flowering plants. It has the lowest saturated fat content of any oil.

Saturated fat is heart-*un*healthy

Cholesterol comes in two forms: "good" cholesterol and "bad." LDL cholesterol (low-density lipoprotein) is the bad one. A diet rich in saturated fat can raise your LDL cholesterol level, which can block healthy blood flow to your heart and brain, increasing your risk of heart disease and stroke. Good cholesterol, called HDL (high-density lipoprotein) cholesterol, acts like a broom, carrying cholesterol away from your arteries and back to your liver for disposal.

Since your body makes saturated fat, you don't need to eat it, but it's hard to avoid, because it's in so many foods—even healthy ones like peanuts and walnuts.

To keep your heart and brain healthy, the American Heart Association says no more than 7% of your total calories should come from saturated fat. That means if you eat 2,000 calories a day, 16 grams of saturated fat is your limit. Eat 9 chicken wings and 1 slice of pepperoni pizza for dinner and you're already there! Two easy ways to put a limit on saturated fat is by eating less cheese and fatty cuts of beef. Here are some other saturated fat-rich foods to avoid or eat only occasionally.

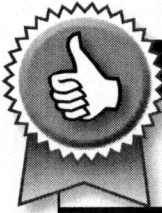

GOOD IDEA!

Strip the skin off your chicken and save 2.5 grams of saturated fat per 3-ounce serving

Saturated Fat-Rich Foods:

- ✧ Fatty cuts of beef, lamb, pork
- ✧ Poultry with skin
- ✧ Lard
- ✧ Cream
- ✧ Butter
- ✧ Cheese

- ✧ Ice Cream
- ✧ Whole milk, 2% milk
- ✧ Bacon
- ✧ Sausage
- ✧ Coconut, palm and palm kernel oils

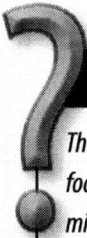

DID YOU KNOW?

The term "fat-free" doesn't necessarily equal "healthy." When fat is removed from a food, it's often replaced with sugar. The number of total calories in a fat-free product might actually be higher than in something that has fat.

The evils of trans fats

Trans fats (trans fatty acids) are created when oil is transformed into solid fat during a process called partial hydrogenation. Commercially baked cakes, cookies and crackers are among the packaged and processed products that contain trans fats. Foods fried in partially hydrogenated oils such as chicken wings and french fries are also high in trans fats. Many

---

? DID YOU KNOW?

Even if a product is labeled "0 grams of trans fat," it can still contain trans fats. Look for the words "partially hydrogenated oil" on the ingredient list. If you spot them, the food is made with trans fat. Put it back on the shelf.

---

food manufacturers and restaurants have done a remarkable job of removing these fats from their products and menus because of their negative health consequences, but beware—trans fats are still hiding out in plenty of products. (Notice the terms *food manufacturers* and *food products*? Just a hundred years ago these words didn't exist. Whenever possible, choose real food made by Mother Nature and unaltered by humans.)

Why is trans fat so dangerous? It raises your total cholesterol and your bad cholesterol levels. If that isn't bad enough, it also lowers your good cholesterol level. In fact, just like saturated fats, trans fats increase your risk of heart disease and stroke.

Your brain hates trans fat, too. It's not natural, so your body doesn't know what to do with it. Not only that, but trans fats don't do any of the good things that natural fats do. Studies have shown that when you eat trans fats, they make their way into your brain cells, interfere with communication between the cells and disrupt your mental performance. Obviously, those are things you want to avoid.

Trans fat is even more harmful than saturated fat. Rather than merely limiting them, it's a good idea to eliminate them from your diet. The American Heart Association recommends that less than 1% of your total calories come from trans fat. This equals 2 grams for a 2,000 calorie diet. Open a bag of Gardetto's Original Recipe Snack Mix and eat one serving and you're already at your limit for the day (a half-cup of the snack mix contains 1.5 grams of trans fat).

Possible Trans Fat-Containing Foods

- Cereals
- Cookies
- Crackers
- Doughnuts
- Foods fried in partially hydrogenated oils: *chicken, french fries, onion rings*
- Frostings
- Margarine
- Microwave popcorn
- Pastry: *pie crusts*
- Potato chips
- Shortening
- Snack cakes
- Snack Mixes
- Tortillas

WARNING! You'll have to do more than look at the nutrition-facts panel to see if a food has trans fat. The FDA requires that trans fats be listed only if the food has 0.5-gram or more per serving. (If you're wondering why some trans fat can be labeled as zero trans fat, you're on your way to discovering that what you read isn't always what you get!) If one of your favorite snack foods contains 0.4-gram of trans fat per serving and you eat it every day, you'll be racking up the trans fats. To tell if a product contains these nasty fats, look at the ingredients list on the food label. If you spot any of the following words, the product contains trans fat:

- ✓ Partially hydrogenated oil
- ✓ Shortening
- ✓ Hydrogenated vegetable oil

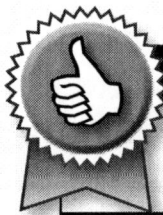

GOOD IDEA!

When buying saltine crackers, choose the Zesta brand for zero grams of trans fats.

Please note that *fully hydrogenated* does not mean trans fat.

Sample of food label with trans fat (labeled as *partially hydrogenated cottonseed oil*)

Ingredients:

ENRICHED FLOUR (WHEAT FLOUR, NIACIN, REDUCED IRON, THIAMINE MONONITRATE (VITAMIN B1), RIBOFLAVIN (VITAMIN B2), FOLIC ACID), SOYBEAN OIL, SALT, HIGH FRUCTOSE CORN SYRUP, **PARTIALLY HYDROGENATED COTTONSEED OIL,** MALTED BARLEY FLOUR, BAKING SODA, VEGETABLE MONOGLYCERIDES (EMULSIFIER).

GOOD IDEA!

While studying for midterms, snack on a handful of peanuts instead of indulging in a couple peanut butter cups.

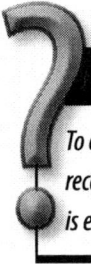

DID YOU KNOW?

To enjoy the benefits of omega 3 fatty acids, the American Heart Association recommends eating 2 servings per week of fatty fish (like salmon or tuna). A serving is equal to 3.5 ounces cooked (about the size of a checkbook, or ¾ cup flaked fish).

Choose brain-building fats

Monounsaturated and polyunsaturated fats are "smart fats." They both lower your total and LDL cholesterol and promote healthy blood flow to your heart and brain. Nuts get a special mention because they're a good source of both these fats and also have vitamin E. Vitamin E is a powerful antioxidant that protects your memory.

Pay special attention to omega 3 fatty acids. They're the building blocks of your brain cells and are considered essential fatty acids. Because your body can't make them, you have to get them from food. Fish has the most "user-friendly" omega 3 fatty acids (in the form of DHA and EPA), but if you don't like it, you can still benefit from non-seafood sources of omega 3's (in the form of ALA) such as walnuts. Studies have shown that EPA and DHA can help stabilize mood and ease depression.

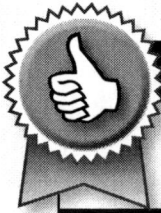

GOOD IDEA!

Choose salmon for dinner instead of a cheeseburger and you're on your way to a healthier brain!

Monounsaturated Fats	Polyunsaturated Fats	
Avocados	Corn oil	
Canola oil	Most nuts and seeds	
Nuts	Safflower oil	
Olive oil	Omega 3 fatty acids:	
Olives		
Peanut oil	***DHA/EPA rich:**	**ALA-rich:**
Seeds	Herring	Omega-3 fatty acid enriched eggs
Sunflower oil	Mackerel	Canola oil — Flaxseed oil
	Salmon	Soybean oil — Chia seeds
	Sardines	Flaxseeds — Pumpkin seeds
	Trout	Soybeans — Tofu
	Tuna	Walnuts

*DHA/EPA-rich fish are listed under "polyunsaturated fats", but should be counted more as a protein (see Secret 5: Lean Your Protein)

DID YOU KNOW?

Some fish, like shark, swordfish, king mackerel or tilefish, contain high levels of mercury, PCBs (polychlorinated biphenyls), dioxins and other environmental contaminants that can be dangerous to your health. Safer fish to eat include: salmon, canned or pouched light tuna, shellfish, pollock and catfish.

SMART-FAT POWER HABITS™!

✓ Replace fried chicken and other breaded and fried foods with grilled or baked ones. Don't forget to remove the skin!

✓ Choose grilled or stir-fried veggies or baked potatoes over french fries.

✓ Read food labels for trans fats! Eliminate foods with partially hydrogenated vegetable oils.

✓ Choose healthier mono and polyunsaturated fats. Grab a small handful of peanuts instead of potato chips or snack mix.

✓ Eat fish twice a week. If you haven't learned to love fish yet, include walnuts or ground flaxseed in your meals and snacks. Mix walnuts into your oatmeal, and sprinkle flaxseed on your salad or mix it into your yogurt.

✓ Limit high-fat dairy products. To save on saturated fat, go for skim or 1% milk instead of 2% or whole. If you eat cheese, keep the portions small (1½ ounces of hard cheese is the size of six stacked dice).

✓ Write your own Smart-Fat Power Habit™: _____

_____

_____

The Bottom Line

Carefully read labels and become aware of the types of fats you're eating. Choose healthier fats when possible. Pick one or two Smart-Fat™ Power Habits from the list above to practice today. Don't forget to record it on your Power Habit™ Tracking Chart in the back of the book!

Secret 3

SHAKE THE SALT

What's in it for you?

✓ Give your diet a one-step extreme makeover

*When you control your sodium,
your entire diet instantly becomes healthier*

Sodium and salt are not the same. Salt is actually sodium chloride and is made up of 40% sodium and 60% chloride. You don't have to worry about getting enough of it, because the average college student eats well over 3,000 mg of sodium every day. Although it's important for your body, eating too much is linked to high blood pressure, heart disease and stroke. Being young and healthy, you might not think you have to worry about disease, but college is the best time to start learning how to prevent it. When you control your sodium, your entire diet instantly becomes healthier.

Recommendations:

✓ Less than 2300 milligrams per day (about 1 teaspoon of salt)

✓ 4700 mg of potassium per day (from food)

Sodium is important in your body for several reasons. It helps to:

✧ Maintain proper fluid balance

✧ Transmit nerve impulses

✧ Contract your muscles

DID YOU KNOW?

Even foods you don't typically think of as being salty contain sodium: Bread has 130 to 170 mg per slice, cereal 140 to 350 mg per serving, instant hot cereal (flavored) 270 mg per packet, and milk 130 mg per cup.

The easiest way to spot a sodium-rich food is to read labels. Certain terms mean less sodium. Choosing these products over their higher-sodium alternatives is one step you can take to shake your salt habit.

Sodium Terminology

✓ Sodium-free: less than 5 mg of sodium per serving

✓ Very low-sodium: 35 mg of sodium or less per serving

✓ Low-sodium: 140 mg of sodium or less per serving

✓ Reduced-sodium: usual sodium level is reduced by 25%

✓ Unsalted, no salt added, without added salt: made without the salt that's normally used, but still contains the sodium that's a natural part of the food

DID YOU KNOW?

Sea salt has just as much sodium as table salt by weight. One teaspoon of sea salt = 2,300 mg of sodium

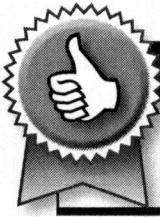

GOOD IDEA!

Instead of ramen noodles, choose a reduced-sodium soup like Campbell's Healthy Request Chicken with Whole Grain Pasta.

If you're eating a cup of ramen noodles for lunch every day, you're probably eating too much sodium. Low-sodium foods such as fruits, vegetables, whole grains and fresh meats will keep you lean, focused and healthy. Think how much better you'll feel and look just by swapping those ramen noodles for a grilled chicken sandwich on whole-grain bread.

Foods High in Sodium	Milligrams of Sodium Per Serving
Canned foods: vegetables, soups, tuna, SpaghettiOs	400-1,400 mg
Condiments: soy sauce, teriyaki sauce, ketchup	190-1,000 mg
Dry packaged convenience foods: soups (ramen noodles), macaroni and cheese	550-1,600 mg
Sauces: marinara	600 mg
Salted pretzels, nuts and potato chips	180-450 mg
Frozen foods: Hot Pockets, frozen dinners	580-1,100 mg
Deli meats	300-1,000 mg
Cheese	175-425 mg
Salad dressings	280-490 mg
Chicken wings in sauce	6 wings = 900 mg
Hot dogs	500 mg
Sausage	800-1,020 mg
Pizza	550-810 mg
Spices containing the word *salt:* garlic salt, seasoning salt	360-490 mg

Uh-oh—eat too much sodium? Let potassium help!

Let's say you couldn't help yourself and went overboard on the Cool Ranch Doritos, polishing off half the bag. Rather than beat yourself up over it, try eating some potassium-rich foods. Potassium has a way of blunting the effects of sodium. Getting the recommended amount of potassium isn't tough to do unless you skip out on fruits and vegetables altogether. Take a look at how quickly those 4,700 mg add up:

Breakfast:	**Potassium (mg):**
1 cup Total Raisin Bran	354
1 cup skim milk	382
1 sliced banana	422

Lunch:	
3 oz. light tuna in water with 1 tbsp olive-oil mayonnaise	201
5 whole-grain crackers	60
1 cup red pepper strips	314
1 cup cantaloupe cubes	160

Dinner:	
3 oz. baked chicken breast	220
1 baked potato	1,081
1 cup broccoli	457
½ cup kidney beans	329

Snack:	
½ cup trail mix with nuts, seeds, chocolate chips and raisins	745

Total potassium:	4,725 mg

Potassium values of various foods can be found at:
http://www.nal.usda.gov/fnic/foodcomp/Data/SR17/wtrank/sr17a306.pdf

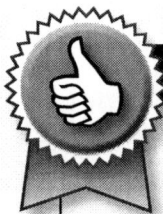

GOOD IDEA!

Frozen dinners can have upwards of 700 mg of sodium per serving. Kashi's Black Bean Mango frozen entrée gets an A+, with only 380 mg of sodium and an impressive 430 mg of potassium and 7 grams of fiber!

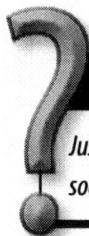

DID YOU KNOW?

Just by switching from regular V8 juice to Low Sodium V8, you can save 280 mg of sodium per 8 ounces.

SALT SHAKIN' POWER HABITS™!

✓ Shelve the salt shaker. Use unsalted spices and herbs to flavor your foods.

✓ Choose lower-sodium soups and snacks.

✓ Eat your fruits and veggies! They're loaded with potassium, which helps blunt sodium's effects on your blood pressure.

✓ Eat fresh or frozen vegetables instead of canned.

✓ If you eat canned foods like beans, vegetables or olives, rinse them under cold water to remove some of the sodium.

✓ Read food labels for sodium!

✓ Eat fewer processed meats like deli meats, hot dogs and sausage and choose more fresh meats like chicken and fish.

✓ Write your own Salt Shakin' Power Habit™: _____

_____

_____

The Bottom Line

Pick one or two Salt Shakin' Power Habits™ from the list above that you can begin doing today and give your diet an instant makeover! Don't forget to record it on your Power Habit™ Tracking Chart in the back of the book!

Secret 4

WHOLE GRAIN
FEEDS YOUR BRAIN

What's in it for you?

✓ Eat less and stay full longer

✓ Get a better night's sleep

✓ Feel happy!

Recommendations:

✓ At least 3 servings of whole grains per day

Love popcorn? Then you must love whole grains!

Y ou've seen the words *whole grain* plastered all over food packages. It's no news that they're good for your health, but do you know why?

Whole grains:

✧ Promote digestive health and prevent constipation

✧ Reduce the risk of heart disease, cancer and diabetes

- ✧ Lower triglycerides (a type of fat found in your blood)
- ✧ Stabilize blood sugar and prevent a "crash and burn" effect in your energy level
- ✧ Help you fight weight gain
- ✧ Fuel your brain

Whole grains are especially good for your brain because they contain carbohydrates that turn into your brain's preferred energy source: glucose. To be sharp, your brain needs a constant supply of glucose. Imagine trying to study all night without energy. It's a lot like trying to drive your car with an empty gas tank.

GOOD IDEA!

Do you love whole-grain rice but hate how long it takes to cook? Minute Rice makes a ready-to-serve whole-grain brown rice that cooks in 1 minute in your microwave.

Honey Vanilla Rice Treat

(280 calories per serving)

1 (4.4-oz. container) Minute Ready to Serve Brown Rice
dash of cinnamon
½ cup low-fat vanilla yogurt
1 tbsp honey
2 tbsp chopped nuts
2 tbsp raisins

Prepare rice according to package directions. Combine cinnamon, yogurt, honey and rice in a small bowl. Stir in nuts and raisins. Makes two servings.
Source: Minuterice.com

Whole grains make you feel happy and calm

After you eat a starchy carbohydrate-rich food like bread, cereal, rice or pasta, the amount of tryptophan in your blood rises. Tryptophan is an amino acid (building block of protein) that your body uses to make serotonin, a powerful brain chemical that:

- ✧ Makes you feel happy and calm
- ✧ Controls your appetite
- ✧ Helps you sleep better
- ✧ Improves your memory
- ✧ Helps you focus, making learning easier
- ✧ Makes you feel energetic

The key is to stick with "smart" carbs, which have nutritional value and aren't too high in sugar—whole-grain bread and crackers are good examples. Choosing carbohydrate-rich foods like soda, candy or cookies will give you a quick energy boost, but within 30 minutes you'll be yawning and heading for Starbucks to make it through the rest of the day or night.

DID YOU KNOW?

Quinoa (pronounced "keen-WAH") is a tiny round grain resembling a sesame seed that is actually a relative of Swiss chard and beets. It is a complete protein because it has all the essential amino acids your body can't make on its own. Quinoa is super-easy to prepare, cooks faster than rice or pasta and makes a great side dish.

What *is* a whole grain?

When you munch on a bowl of popcorn while watching your favorite movie, you may not realize that you're actually indulging in a bowl of whole grains! It's really not hard to meet the minimum recommendations for whole grains when you know what they are. Unlike refined grains, whole grains contain the entire grain kernel: the bran, endosperm and germ.

DID YOU KNOW?

Just because a food package says "whole grain" or "made with whole grain" doesn't mean it's a true whole grain. Check the first word under the list of ingredients and if it's "whole", it's most likely a whole grain.

When a whole grain is put through the refining process, two of the layers are stripped off, along with 17 key nutrients, fiber and a good portion of protein.

The fiber in whole grains slows its digestion, releasing a steady stream of glucose to your brain. Let's say you eat a bowl of Rice Krispies for breakfast. Even though it may be enriched with vitamins and minerals, it's still a refined grain with little fiber. Don't be surprised if you're hungry again in an hour. Eat a bowl of Cheerios, or better yet oatmeal, and you'll be satisfied for a few hours.

B-vitamins turn the energy from the food you eat into energy you can use. Without them, getting through your day would be a lot harder. Whole grains are a great source of B-vitamins, another good reason to make them a staple in your diet.

GOOD IDEA!

The next time you have a taste for cheese and crackers, reach for Triscuits or Kashi Heart to Heart Crackers. Both are whole-grain!

DID YOU KNOW?

White whole wheat bread is considered a whole grain because it is made from the entire grain kernel. The only difference between white whole wheat and regular whole wheat bread is the type of wheat. White whole wheat comes from white wheat and has a softer texture, while traditional whole wheat comes from red wheat. Both are equally nutritious.

You can tell if a grain is a whole grain by checking the food label. If the first ingredient is one of the following, it's a whole grain:

Whole Grain Terminology

- ✧ Amaranth*
- ✧ Barley
- ✧ Brown Rice*
- ✧ Buckwheat*
- ✧ Bulgur
- ✧ Corn*
- ✧ Kamut
- ✧ Millet*
- ✧ Oatmeal (including instant)
- ✧ Popcorn
- ✧ Oats
- ✧ Quinoa*
- ✧ Rye
- ✧ Sorghum*
- ✧ Spelt
- ✧ Stoneground whole (name of grain)
- ✧ Wheatberries
- ✧ Whole (name of grain)
- ✧ Whole grain
- ✧ Whole wheat
- ✧ Wild Rice*

Gluten-free grains

Here are two food labels for bread. One is a whole grain and the other is not.

Refined bread	Whole grain bread
Ingredients: Enriched Flour (Wheat Flour, Malt Barley Flour, Niacin, Ferrous Sulfate, Thiamine Mononitrate, Riboflavin, Folic Acid), Water, High Fructose Corn Syrup, Yeast, Soy Oil, Contains 2% or less of the following: Salt, Mono-Diglycerides, Mono Calcium Phosphate, Calcium Sulfate, Calcium Propionate (A Preservative), Ammonium Sulfate, Enzyme, Ascorbic Acid, Azodicarbonamide (ADA), Calcium Peroxide, Soy Lecithin.	**Ingredients: Whole Wheat Flour,** Water, Whole Wheat, Vital Wheat Gluten, Brown Sugar, Whole Rye, Yeast, Honey, Molasses, Soybean Oil, Salt, Cultured Wheat Flour, Yeast Nutrients (Ammonium Sulfate, Monocalcium Phosphate), Dough Conditioners (Malted Barley Flour, Calcium Sulfate, Enzymes), Niacin, Ferrous Sulfate (Iron), Thiamine Mononitrate (Vitamin B1), Riboflavin (Vitamin B2), and Folic Acid, Soy Lecithin.

DID YOU KNOW?

Unless it's specifically labeled as whole-grain bread, choosing wheat, multigrain or 12-grain bread for your sandwich is just like asking for white bread. They all lack the entire grain kernel. Buy whole wheat or whole grain and ask for these when you order toast or a sandwich at a restaurant.

What counts as a serving?

You should aim for at least three servings of whole grains every day. Each of the following contains one serving of whole grain.

Whole Grain Food	Example	Serving Size
Whole grain bread	100% Whole Wheat Wonder Bread	1 slice
Whole grain bagel	Thomas' Hearty Grains 100% Whole Wheat Bagels	½ of a medium or 1 mini bagel (1 large bagel = 4 servings)
Whole grain cereal	Cheerios	1 cup
Crackers	Kashi Heart to Heart Crackers	About 5
English Muffin	Thomas' 100% Whole Wheat English Muffins	½ of a muffin
Hot cereal	Quaker Oatmeal	½ cup cooked
Pasta, rice, or other grain	Barilla Whole Grain Pasta	½ cup cooked
Popcorn	Smart Balance Smart 'n Healthy Popcorn	3 cups popped
Tortilla	Mission Yellow Corn Tortillas	1 small (6" diameter)

CAUTION: Beware of foods with these words on the package:

✓ "Made with whole grain"
✓ "Multigrain"
✓ "12 grain"
✓ "Wheat"

Although they sound impressive, if the first word on the ingredient list isn't one from the whole-grain table above, you won't be eating a whole grain. Put it back on the shelf and look for a true whole-grain product. They aren't hard to find. In the appendix you'll find a grocery list that includes many recommended whole-grain products.

GOOD IDEA!

Eat a slice of whole-grain toast with your breakfast, a Kashi TLC Roasted Almond Crunch granola bar as an afternoon snack and a small bowl of Raisin Bran before you go to bed. Guess what—you've just met the minimum recommendations for whole grain!

Look for the whole-grain stamp

Thanks to a nonprofit group called the Whole Grains Council, it's easier than ever to spot a true whole-grain product. The council created the official Whole Grain Stamp, which started appearing on products in 2005.

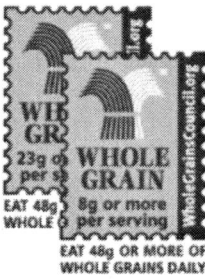

THE BASIC STAMP

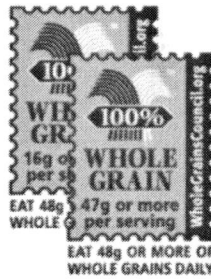

THE 100% STAMP

The Basic Stamp:	The 100% Stamp:
✧ The product may contain some extra bran, germ or refined flour ✧ Minimum requirement: 8 grams whole grain per serving (half-serving of whole grain) Source: www.wholegrainscouncil.org	✧ All the grain is a whole grain ✧ Minimum requirement: 16 grams whole grain per serving (a full serving of whole grain)

Not all whole-grain products have the stamp, however, only those whose manufacturers are members of the Whole Grains Council. Brands in the council include:

Aladdin Baking Company	Healthy Choice	Ronzoni
Bagel Bites	Heartland	Ry Krisp
Barilla	Hungry Jack	Sara Lee
Arrowhead Mills	Kashi	Schwebel's
Aunt Millie's Hearth	Kellogg	Smucker's
Back to Nature	Kroger	Snyder's of Hanover
Bear Naked	Lean Pockets	Sunbelt
Brownberry	Lender's	SunChips
Bob's Red Mill	Minute Rice	Thomas
Cascadian Farm	Nature's Own	Tony's Pizza
Corazonas Foods	Nature's Path	Tostitos
Cream of Wheat	Nickles Bakery	Trader Joe's
Country Hearth	Old El Paso	Tyson Foods
Dr. Kracker	Ortega	Uncle Ben's
Fiber One	Otis Spunkmeyer	Vitalicious
Fieldstone	Perdue	Wal-Mart
Garden of Eatin'	Pillsbury	Weight Watchers Whole
General Mills	Post	Foods Market Wonder Bread
Giant Eagle	Quaker Oats Company	
Health Valley	Roman Meal	

To check if your favorite product is wearing the stamp, visit the Whole Grains Council at: http://www.wholegrainscouncil.org/find-whole-grains/stamped-products.

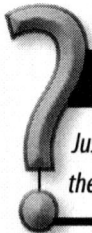

DID YOU KNOW?

Just because a product has a load of fiber doesn't mean it's a true whole grain. Read the list of ingredients to be sure.

WHOLE GRAIN POWER HABITS™!

✓ Go whole grain! When choosing bread, cereal or pasta, be sure the first word on the list of ingredients is "whole".

✓ Visit the Whole Grains Council and look for your favorite cereal or granola bar. www.wholegrainscouncil.org

✓ Choose brown rice instead of white rice.

✓ Eat a bowl of oatmeal for breakfast.

✓ Snack on whole grain chips like SunChips instead of potato chips.

✓ Order your sandwich or wrap on whole grain bread or in a whole grain tortilla.

✓ Toss a whole grain cereal bar like Kashi Honey Almond & Flax into your bag for a quick snack between classes.

✓ Write your own Whole Grain Power Habit™: _____

_____

_____

The Bottom Line

Whole grains are healthier than refined ones. Go whole grain today by picking one or two Whole Grain Power Habits™ above. Don't forget to record it on your Power Habit™ Tracking Chart in the back of the book!

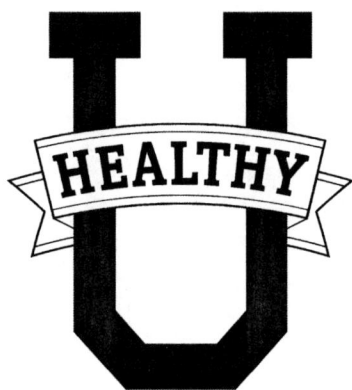

Secret 5

LEAN YOUR PROTEIN

What's in it for you?

✓ Stay full longer

✓ Have more energy

✓ Make studying easier

✓ Be alert in your classes

✓ Improve concentration for exams

Recommendations:

✓ 5-7 ounces of lean protein daily (based on a 2,000 calorie diet)

✓ 2 servings of omega 3 fatty acid-rich fish a week

Chances are you don't need as much protein as you think

For peak mental focus and energy, you need protein. It'll also help you feel full longer, a good way to avoid unhealthy snacks and sidestep college weight gain. A bowl of oatmeal for breakfast is a wise choice, but you'll be more alert and satisfied if you have an egg on the side. You'll definitely feel the difference!

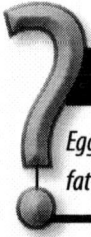

Eat protein and stay awake in class

Protein contains essential and nonessential amino acids. An essential amino acid is critical for human health but can't be manufactured in the body. Complete proteins like meat, poultry, fish, milk, eggs and cheese have all nine essential amino acids.

A little protein with your breakfast, such as a tablespoon of peanut butter on your toast, and a protein-rich lunch like a tuna fish sandwich on whole-grain bread raise the level of the amino acid tyrosine in your blood. Dopamine, epinephrine and norepinephrine, the "fight or flight" chemicals in your body, are made from tyrosine and help you to:

✓ Respond well to stress

✓ Be alert

✓ Stay focused and energized

Who knew a tuna fish sandwich could not only help you stay awake during class but keep you focused, too?

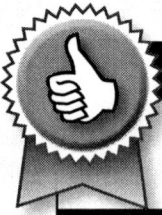

GOOD IDEA!

Instead of snacking on a plain banana, try it with a tablespoon of nut butter. Peanut, almond and cashew butters are all delicious and healthy

Be smart—choose lean proteins

When it comes to the source of protein in your diet, opt for lean protein, including fish. Because it's high in brain-building omega 3 fatty acids, the American Heart Association recommends eating two servings of fatty fish like salmon, light tuna, mackerel, herring or trout every week.

All these fish have low or moderate mercury levels. The table below lists great sources of lean proteins.

Leaner Proteins	Portion Size
Beans and legumes	¼ cup
Eggs	1 egg
Fish	3 oz. (size of a checkbook)
Hummus	2 tablespoons
Lean cuts of beef or pork: Look for "loin" or "round" cuts, and choose "choice" or "select" grades of beef	3 oz. (size of a deck of cards)
Nuts and seeds Nut butters: peanut butter, almond butter	½ oz. 1 tablespoon
Soy: Soybeans Tofu Soy burger	 ¼ cup ¼ cup 1 burger = 2 oz.
Turkey and chicken: skinless white meat (breast)	3 oz. (size of a deck of cards)

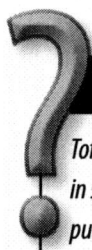

DID YOU KNOW?

Tofu is a meat substitute made from soybean curd, a soft cheese-like protein. It comes in silken and firm textures. Silken is more like a custard and is used in blended or pureed dishes, while firm is sponge-like and can be stir-fried or grilled.

To cut down on saturated fat and sodium:

Eat more often:	Eat less often:
Grilled Broiled Baked Roasted Poached Stir-fried	Fried Breaded Deep-fried Meats in heavy cream Meats covered in gravy Processed meats: ham, sausage, hot dogs, deli meats

GOOD IDEA!

Add some edamame to your tuna salad for a different flavor and added nutrition.

Tuna Edamame Salad:

(210 calories per 1-cup serving)

½ cup edamame, cooked according to package directions
½ cup cherry tomatoes, cut in half
½ cup shredded carrots
3-oz can of low-sodium light tuna, drained
¼ cup golden raisins
2 tbsp diced red onion
2 tbsp bottled Italian salad dressing

Mix edamame, tomatoes, carrots, tuna, raisins and onion in a medium bowl. Pour dressing over salad and toss until combined. Serve with pita bread halves or whole-grain crackers, if desired.
Makes 2 servings.
Source: Soyconnection.com

DID YOU KNOW?

Hummus is a thick dip made from mashed chickpeas (also called garbanzo beans or cece beans) and tahini (sesame-seed paste). There are many varieties, and it's much more nutritious than ranch dressing or mayonnaise.

Still aren't convinced that you need to lean your protein? Take a look at the side-by-side comparison of a McDonald's cheeseburger, KFC grilled chicken breast and grilled salmon.

Nutrition Facts	McDonald's Cheeseburger (4 oz.)	KFC Grilled Chicken Breast (4 oz.)	Grilled Salmon (4 oz.)
Calories	300	210	244
Fat	12 grams	8 grams	12.4 grams
Saturated fat	6 grams	2.5 grams	2.2 grams
Trans fat	0.5-gram	0	0
Sodium	750 mg	460 mg	75 mg
Protein	15 grams	34 grams	31 grams

KFC's Grilled Chicken Breast and grilled salmon are the definite winners, cashing in at twice the protein and fewer calories than the burger.

At first glance you might think the cheeseburger is a better choice than salmon because it's lower in total fat. But the amount of saturated fat is more important than the total fat. The salmon is only 8% saturated fat, while the cheeseburger is 18% saturated fat (with an additional 0.5-gram of trans fat). Saturated and trans fats are the bad ones. The fat in salmon is the brain-building omega 3 fat, the one you want to load up on.

Eating a cheeseburger once in a while won't kill you, but how often do you order just a cheeseburger? How often do you choose the Angus Deluxe instead of a single burger with one slice of cheese? Take a look at how this measures up.

Nutrition Facts	McDonald's Angus Deluxe (11.1 oz.)
Calories	750
Fat	39 grams
Saturated fat	16 grams (19%)
Trans fat	2 grams
Sodium	1,700 mg (74%)
Protein	40 grams

Don't lose your head at the deli counter

Ok, let's be honest. As a college student, you will no doubt be faced

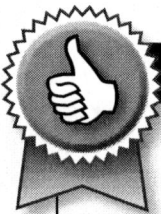

GOOD IDEA!

If you like the convenience of deli meats, try a lower-sodium version like Sara Lee's Lower Sodium Oven Roasted Chicken Breast. Although it's still a higher-sodium food (350 mg of sodium in a 2-ounce portion), it sure beats Oscar Mayer's Oven Roasted Chicken Breast (700 mg of sodium in a 2-ounce portion).

with sub sandwiches piled high with cold cuts like ham and turkey. Processed meats are salted, smoked, cured or preserved with nitrates. Hot dogs, sausage, salami, ham, bacon, deli cold cuts, pepperoni and other cured meats typically contain lots of salt and fat. Before you order a Spicy Italian sub from Subway, digest the following facts about processed meats:

✓ According to a 2010 news release from the National Cancer Institute, researchers found that eating high amounts of processed red meats leads to increased risk of bladder cancer.

✓ Eating processed meats can raise your risk of heart disease and diabetes.

✓ Two ounces of processed meat can have as much as 700 mg of sodium.

It's okay to eat a lunch-meat sandwich once in a while, but be smart and choose fresh-meat subs most often.

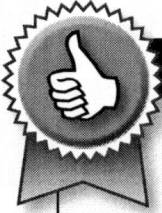

GOOD IDEA!

For a quick protein pick-me-up, keep a box of Spicy Black Bean Burgers by MorningStar Farms in your freezer. One patty has only 120 calories but offers 11 grams of protein, 4 grams of fat (only 0.5 saturated) and 4 grams of fiber. It takes only a few minutes to cook in your toaster oven or a skillet with a touch of canola oil, or pop it in the microwave for 1 minute. Eat it plain on a whole-grain bun.

LEAN PROTEIN POWER HABITS™!

✓ Opt for grilled, baked, poached, broiled or roasted meats, and go easy on the sauces.

✓ Go fish for a powerful brain! Try it just one time a week for starters.

✓ Combine your carbohydrates with lean protein for maximum energy and focus.

✓ Choose more fresh-meat sandwiches and fewer deli meats.

✓ Snacks need protein, too. Instead of a handful of baby carrots, how about adding a hard-boiled egg or a handful of nuts or seeds on the side?

✓ Try soybeans on your salad or a soy burger for lunch.

✓ Write your own Lean Protein Power Habit™: _____

_____

_____

The Bottom Line

The source of protein in your diet and how it's prepared matters. Start small by choosing one or two of the Lean Protein Power Habits™ above. Don't forget to record it on your Power Habit™ Tracking Chart in the back of the book!

Secret 6

BANK ON CALCIUM

What's in it for you?

✓ Build strong bones now, while you can

✓ Ease PMS

Daily Recommendations:

✓ 17- and 18-year-olds: 1,300 mg (4 cups of milk or milk equivalents) plus 600 IU vitamin D

✓ 19 and older: 1,000 mg (3 cups of milk or milk equivalents) plus 600 IU vitamin D

At age 30, your bones will have reached peak bone mass

According to the USDA's Continuing Survey of Food Intakes by Individuals, more than 85% of female college students and 67% of male students don't get enough calcium. How are you supposed to prevent osteoporosis later in life if you aren't building a strong bone foundation in your late teens and early twenties?

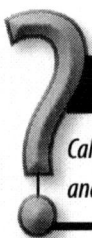

DID YOU KNOW?

Calcium makes up 1.5% to 2% of your body weight, and 99% of it is in your bones and teeth.

I didn't care much for milk when I was a college student, so I'd walk to the local coffee shop every day and order a large cappuccino made with skim milk. It got expensive, but at least I was getting my calcium!

—MELANIE JATSEK, University of Akron graduate

Your body on calcium

Your bones and teeth rely on calcium to keep them strong, along with vitamin D to help absorb it. Now is the time to invest in your "bone bank" because once you hit age 30, your bones will have reached peak bone mass. At that point, you can't make any more deposits.

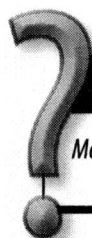

DID YOU KNOW?

Men can (and do) suffer from osteoporosis, too.

Calcium plays a role in contracting and expanding your muscles and blood vessels and offers relief from premenstrual syndrome (PMS). Research has shown that women who get the recommended amount of calcium (1,000 to 1,300 mg) every day enjoy relief from the majority of PMS symptoms, including cramping and irritability. So, during that time of the month, women, pour a nice tall glass of skim milk for yourself. And men, you might want to pour some for your girlfriends!

Low-fat milk and yogurt are great sources of calcium, protein and carbohydrates, making them the perfect foods to re-energize your body after a rigorous workout. The carbohydrates replenish your energy while the protein rebuilds your muscles. Cheese has calcium, fat and protein but very few (if any) carbohydrates.

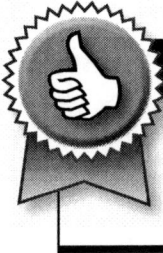

GOOD IDEA!

For a real calcium boost, top your baked potato with low-fat yogurt instead of sour cream. Or better yet, try a fresh green juice made with kale or spinach.

What counts as a serving?

Milk & Milk Equivalents	Serving Size	Calcium (mg)
Cow's milk (skim)	8 oz.	300
Natural cheese: Cheddar, mozzarella, Swiss	1½ oz.	200-330
Shredded cheese	1/3 cup	200-300
Yogurt (plain, low-fat)	8 oz.	400

Non-Dairy Sources of Calcium	Serving Size	Calcium (mg)
Blackstrap molasses	1 tablespoon	172
Calcium-fortified cereals (e.g., Total)	1 oz.	100-1000
Calcium-fortified juices	8 oz.	100-350
Calcium-fortified soy, almond, or rice milk	8 oz.	300
Calcium-set tofu (firm, extra-firm)	½ cup	100-860
Collard greens, cooked	1 cup	300
Fish with bones	3 oz.	180-300
Kale, cooked	1 cup	94

Non-Dairy Sources of Calcium	Serving Size	Calcium (mg)
Spinach, cooked	1 cup	245
Soybeans	½ cup	130
Turnip greens, cooked	1 cup	200

Source: National Institutes of Health-Office of Dietary Supplements

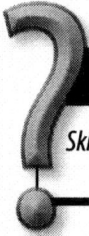

DID YOU KNOW?

Skim and 1% milk have more calcium than 2% and whole milk.

Top 10 Calcium-Containing Cereals

All values are for one serving according to nutrition facts on package

1. *Total Whole Grain: 1,000 mg*
2. *Total Raisin Bran: 1,000 mg*
3. *Total Honey Almond Flax: 1,000 mg*
4. *Quaker True Delights Instant Oatmeal: 250 mg*
5. *Cream of Wheat: 200 mg*
6. *Kix: 150 mg*
7. *Fiber One: 100 mg*
8. *Cheerios: 100 mg*
9. *Life: 100 mg*
10. *Cascadian Farms Fruitful O's: 100 mg*

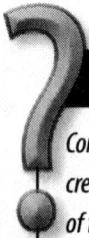

DID YOU KNOW?

Compared to regular yogurt, Greek yogurt is higher in protein and lower in sugar, creamier and will keep you full longer. Some varieties can have as much as 23 grams of fat per 8 ounces, so choose the fat-free or 2% fat varieties.

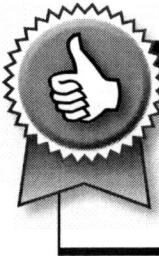

GOOD IDEA!

Have a bowl of Total cereal (1,000 mg calcium) with 8 ounces of skim milk (300 mg calcium) for breakfast and you've reached your calcium goal for the day!

The skinny on dairy

You've learned that diets high in saturated fat raise your risk for heart disease and stroke, so before you decide to dig into an ice cream sundae or a plate of cheese-drenched nachos, keep in mind that these full-fat dairy products are also laden with saturated fat. Take a look at the saturated-fat content of some high-fat dairy products and compare them with some healthier alternatives.

Instead of these saturated fat-rich dairy products	Grams of saturated fat	Choose these healthier dairy products	Grams of saturated fat
Cheddar cheese (1 oz.)	6 grams	Mozzarella cheese (1 oz.)	3.7 grams
Ice cream (1 cup)	9 grams	Low-fat yogurt (6 oz.)	0-2 grams
Whole milk (1 cup)	4.5 grams	1% milk (1 cup)	1.5 grams
2% milk (1 cup)	3.1 grams	Skim milk (1 cup)	0-0.5 gram

Source: USDA Nutrient Data Laboratory

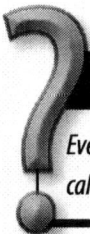

DID YOU KNOW?

Even though a cookie-dough Blizzard from Dairy Queen has an impressive 350 mg of calcium, it also has a shocking 16 grams of saturated fat—and that's the small size!

Remember vitamin D:

If you want to absorb calcium, you need vitamin D. It's known as the "sunshine vitamin" because your body makes it after being exposed to sunshine—all it takes is spending a short time outside in direct sunlight (about 5-30 minutes) two to three times a week to make enough vitamin D. But this can be a challenge if you go to school in a state without a year-round sunny climate. Food sources of vitamin D include:

Food Sources of Vitamin D	Serving Size	Vitamin D (IU)
Cereal	1 cup	40 or more
Cod liver oil	1 tablespoon	1,360
Eggs, large	1 yolk	41
Milk	8 oz.	115-124
Salmon	3 oz.	447
Tuna	3 oz.	154
Vitamin D-fortified orange juice	8 oz.	100
Yogurt	6 oz.	80

Source: National Institutes of Health Office of Dietary Supplements

To supplement or not to supplement?

If you're one of the many college students not getting enough of this important mineral, you may want to consider a calcium supplement. They come in two forms: calcium citrate and calcium carbonate. Your body absorbs calcium citrate equally effectively when taken with or without food, whereas calcium carbonate is best absorbed *with* food. It's a good idea to cap the calcium at 500 mg at a time because your body does a better job absorbing it in limited doses. Viactiv Calcium Chews are a great-tasting option, supplying 500 mg of calcium in the form of calcium carbonate and 500 IU of vitamin D.

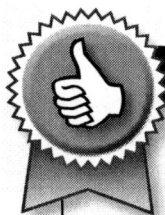

GOOD IDEA!

Yogurt doesn't have to be boring. Try making your own "cereal sundae" by mixing your favorite low-fat yogurt, cereal and fruit!

Cereal Sundae:

(460 calories and 40% DV for calcium)

1 cup of your favorite low-fat yogurt

½ cup of your favorite whole grain cereal

½ cup of your favorite fresh or frozen fruit (use canned if it's easier; pineapple and mandarin oranges work well)

Mix yogurt, cereal and fruit in a bowl or a tall glass and enjoy!
Makes one serving.

What if you can't tolerate milk?

Do you ever experience diarrhea or feel bloated or gassy after drinking a glass of milk? You may be lactose intolerant.

Lactose is the natural sugar in milk that some people can't digest, leading to these unwelcome side effects. If this sounds like you, it may be difficult for you to get enough calcium in your diet. Here are a few tips to help:

✓ Drink milk in smaller portions (4 ounces or less) and with food. This can sometimes scale back the side effects.

✓ Try lactose-free milk such as Lactaid, Dairy Ease or calcium-fortified soy milk.

✓ Try aged cheeses like cheddar and Swiss. They have low lactose levels and may be tolerated.

✓ Yogurt contains live active cultures that aid in the digestion of lactose, so you might do fine with it.

✓ If you're still gassy and bloated, try adding more non-dairy sources of calcium to your diet such as soybeans and calcium-fortified juices.

BONE-BANKING POWER HABITS™!

✓ If you don't like plain milk, blend 1% or skim milk with fruit and yogurt for a calcium-loaded smoothie.

✓ Eat string cheese for your afternoon snack.

✓ For a great midmorning snack, stir a small handful of peanuts and low-fat granola into a container of your favorite low-fat yogurt.

✓ Make it skinny! Order your latte or mocha with skim milk instead of 2% or whole milk.

✓ Use milk instead of water when making pancakes, oatmeal or Cream of Wheat.

✓ Write you our own Bone-Banking Power Habit™: _____

_____

_____

The Bottom Line

If you don't build healthy bones now, you'll regret it later. Track your calcium servings today to see if you're getting enough. If not, what Bone-Banking Power Habits™ will you choose to incorporate from the list above? Don't forget to record it on your Power Habit™ Tracking Chart in the back of the book!

Secret 7

FEED YOUR SWEET TOOTH WITH FRUIT

What's in it for you?

✓ Break your sugar addiction

✓ Keep the pounds off

✓ Stay full longer

✓ Get and stay focused

✓ Avoid your yearly cold

Recommendations:

✓ 1½ to 2 cups of fruit per day

When was the last time you tossed a handful of M&M's into your mouth for a quick pick-me-up? That's exactly what you end up getting when you snack on sweets, a quick pick-me-up—followed by a "crash and burn" effect. Not exactly what you had in mind, right?

Sweets have a place in a healthy diet—a small place

GOOD IDEA!

Turn your oatmeal into a healthy slice of apple pie without the guilt!

Oatmeal Apple Pie:

(300 calories)

½ cup dry oatmeal

1 cup water

1 small apple with skin, diced

7 walnut halves

1 tsp unpacked brown sugar

dash of cinnamon

Put all ingredients in a microwave-safe bowl. Microwave for 90 seconds. Top with cinnamon and enjoy!

Sugar Digestion 101:

You've learned that your brain relies on a constant supply of carbohydrates (in the form of glucose) to be at its sharpest. Sugar is a quickly digesting carbohydrate, so when you eat or drink a sugary food or beverage like M&M's or soda, your pancreas gets a signal to produce insulin. Insulin triggers your cells to "mop up" the glucose and store it for later use. That's what a healthy body is supposed to do. The problem is, soon your blood-sugar levels start to plummet and you're left crashing and burning with no energy and a foggy brain.

So what's the answer? Do you swear off sugar for the rest of your life? Should you pass up your favorite sweet treats from here to eternity? Of course not! They have their place in a balanced diet, but probably a much smaller place than you're used to. That's why it's important to know which carbohydrates are "brain building" and which are "brain draining".

? DID YOU KNOW?

Eating too much sugar will not cause diabetes. Eating too much of any food (including sugary foods) can make you gain weight, however, and being overweight is one of the main risk factors for developing type 2 diabetes.

Brain-building and brain-draining carbohydrates

Brain-building carbohydrates are like capsules. When you take a pain-relief capsule like Tylenol, it breaks down slowly, releasing a steady steam of its contents into your bloodstream. That's exactly how brain-building carbohydrates digest. You'll be much more alert and focused in class if you eat a whole-grain bagel for breakfast instead of a blueberry muffin. Brain-building carbohydrates include:

✔ Whole-grain cereals, crackers, bread, pasta, oats, brown rice, etc.

✔ Fruit (fresh or frozen rather than juice)

✔ Legumes: dried beans, peas and lentils

✔ Milk and yogurt

✔ Vegetables

Brain-draining carbohydrates, on the other hand, are refined foods made from white flour and added sugars. Eating that blueberry muffin for breakfast is sort of like taking a syringe and injecting the carbohydrate right into your vein for immediate glucose. Brain-draining carbohydrates include:

✔ White bread, bagels

✔ Muffins, pastries, doughnuts

✔ White rice

✔ Sugary cereals

✔ Cookies

✔ Cakes

✓ Candy

✓ Frosting

✓ Kool-Aid and fruit drinks

✓ Soda

✓ Sweetened coffee drinks

✓ Sweet tea

✓ Sweeteners: table sugar, syrups, jams, jellies, brown sugar, raw sugar

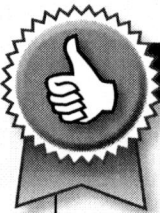

GOOD IDEA!

If you're dying for a Krispy Kreme donut, try a Super Donut instead! You can find them in the frozen-foods section of your grocery store. One Super Donut has 180 calories, 5 grams of fat (1.5 saturated), 5 grams of protein and 14 vitamins and minerals, including calcium and vitamin D.

Read food labels to spot a potential brain-draining carbohydrate. If any of the following ingredients are listed on the label, the product has added sugars.

Ingredients that equal added sugars

- ◈ Brown sugar
- ◈ Corn sweetener
- ◈ Corn syrup
- ◈ Dextrose
- ◈ Fructose
- ◈ Fruit-juice concentrates
- ◈ Glucose
- ◈ High-fructose corn syrup
- ◈ Honey
- ◈ Invert sugar
- ◈ Lactose
- ◈ Maltose
- ◈ Malt syrup
- ◈ Molasses
- ◈ Raw sugar
- ◈ Sucrose
- ◈ Sugar
- ◈ Syrup

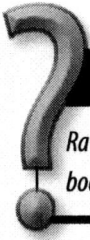

DID YOU KNOW?

Raw sugar, brown sugar and honey are no healthier than white table sugar. Your body digests them all the same way.

Here's how your favorite sugary foods and beverages stack up in terms of sugar:

Your favorite sugary foods and beverages	Grams of sugar	Equals this many teaspoons of sugar
12-oz. soda	42	10.5
Chocolate bar (1.5 oz)	24	6
Grande Caffé Mocha	32	8
3 cream-filled chocolate cookies	14	3.5
Cereal (Trix)	13	3.25
¼ cup pancake syrup	32	8
1 tablespoon jam or jelly	12	3
8 oz. of juice	26	6.5
1 can of energy drink (8.5 oz)	27.5	7
1 teaspoon of table sugar	4.2	1
½ cup chocolate ice cream	16	4

In Secret 4, you learned that eating healthy carbohydrate-rich foods raises the level of tryptophan in your body, which makes serotonin and in turn leaves you happy, calm and in control of your appetite. When you snack on sugary foods, the effect is quite different. Don't be surprised if you're a bit moody and sluggish after digging into a bag of Tootsie Rolls while studying for your chemistry exam. If you're craving something sweet and have a long night of cramming ahead, eat a cluster of grapes or a handful of raisins instead.

Boycott most sugar substitutes

Soft drinks, yogurt, chewing gum, cereal, jelly, candy and ice cream are just a few of the products made with sugar substitutes. You may see them labeled as "sugar-free" or "diet." They fall into two categories: artificial sweeteners and sugar alcohols.

Artificial sweeteners:

Artificial sweeteners are hundreds to thousands of times sweeter than white table sugar and can actually increase your craving for sugar. Surprisingly, several large studies have shown a link between artificial-sweetener use and weight gain! Those artificial sweeteners approved by the FDA are:

✓ Acesulfame potassium (Sunett, Sweet One)

✓ Aspartame (Equal, NutraSweet)

✓ Neotame

✓ Saccharin (SugarTwin, Sweet'N Low)

✓ Sucralose (Splenda)

Sugar alcohols:

Sugar alcohols are made from carbohydrates, not alcohol. They aren't any sweeter than sugar, but they do have fewer calories. You can't go to the store and pick up a box of sugar alcohols because they're found only in certain processed foods and food products.

To spot an FDA-approved sugar alcohol, look for any of the following words on the list of ingredients:

✓ Erythritol

✓ Hydrogenated starch hydrolysates

✓ Isomalt

✓ Lactitol

✓ Maltitol

✓ Mannitol

✓ Sorbitol

✓ Xylitol

✓ Stevia preparations that are highly refined (Pure Via, Truvia)

Sugar alcohols can have a laxative-type effect, causing gas, bloating and diarrhea in certain people, so use them in moderation.

The big question on the minds of many college students is, "If I'm trying to watch my weight, isn't it better to eat foods with artificial sweeteners than foods with sugar?" Unless you have a condition like diabetes, where too much sugar will cause your blood-sugar levels to become dangerously high, the answer is no. There really is no reason to choose a diet yogurt over a regular one. Of course, you'll still want to read the label for grams of sugar and choose the foods with the least amount possible.

As with regular sugar, if you eat foods made with sugar substitutes, be smart and don't overindulge. Just because a food is labeled "sugar-free" doesn't mean it's calorie-free.

I used to buy everything sugar-free. I thought I was doing a good thing by saving on calories, but I slowly began to realize that I was eating more! It wasn't until I put a limit on the artificial sweeteners and began eating more "real" food that I noticed how good "real" food could be, and my appetite slowed down too. Now when I eat or drink something with artificial sweeteners, I can't even finish it, because it just doesn't taste good. It's too sweet!

—AMANDA, the University of Texas at Austin

Why fruit?

Fruits are rich in potassium, fiber, folate, vitamin C and beta-carotene (a precursor to vitamin A). Vitamin C and beta-carotene are powerful antioxidants, natural substances in foods that clean up free radicals in your body. We all have free radicals floating around inside our bodies. They are formed as a byproduct of reactions in your cells and also come from cigarette smoke, air pollution and exposure to ultraviolet (UV) rays. In toxic amounts, they cause damage to your body, loss of brain function over time and are believed to be a main contributor to heart disease, certain cancers and Parkinson's disease. So it's important to get rid of as many of them as possible. Your body does a pretty good job, but it can't remove them all. That's why you need to eat fruits and vegetables every day. Berries have the highest antioxidant power of any fruit, so choose them whenever possible.

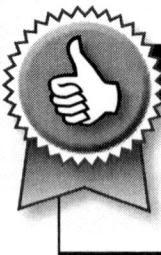

GOOD IDEA!

Make your own trail mix with your favorite dried fruit, nuts and cereal. Figs, apricots, raisins and prunes have the most potassium. Just keep your portions small.

Top-Scoring Antioxidant-Rich Fruits

(Source: USDA Database for the Oxygen Radical Absorbance Capacity (ORAC) of Selected Foods, May 2010)

✧ Apples with skins	✧ Figs	✧ Peaches
✧ Apricots (dried)	✧ Grapefruit	✧ Pears
✧ Avocados	✧ Grapes	✧ Plums/prunes
✧ Berries	✧ Guava	✧ Pomegranates
✧ Cherries	✧ Kiwi	✧ Raisins
✧ Currants	✧ Oranges	✧ Mangoes

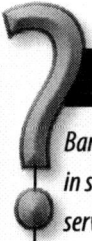

DID YOU KNOW?

Banana chips don't count as a fruit serving. They are typically deep-fried and coated in sugar or honey, packing a whopping 10 grams of fat (9 saturated) per half-cup serving. Eat a regular banana instead for 0 grams of fat.

Vitamin C and beta-carotene strengthen your immune system, too, so you'll be less likely to get sick during finals week when you make fruit a regular part of your diet.

Beta-Carotene-Rich Fruits	Vitamin C-Rich Fruits
Apricots	Berries
Cantaloupe	Cantaloupe
Cherries	Grapefruit
Mangoes	Honeydew
Nectarines	Kiwi
Peaches	Mangoes
Pink grapefruit	Nectarines
Tangerines	Oranges
Watermelon	Papaya
	Strawberries

For the most protection, try to eat 1½ to two cups of fruit a day. One cup of fruit is equal to:

✓ 1 medium pear or grapefruit

✓ 1 large banana, peach or orange

✓ 1 small apple

✓ ½ cup dried fruit

✓ 1 standard measuring cup of any fruit (such as pineapple chunks, berries, grapes and diced cantaloupe, honeydew and watermelon)

? DID YOU KNOW?

Frozen fruit is affordable and just as nutritious (if not more so) as fresh fruit because it's flash-frozen immediately after harvesting to preserve the nutrients. Just be sure it doesn't have added sugars.

Notice that 100% fruit juice is not on this list. Although it's a natural sugar and has more nutrition than soda, it still has lots of sugar. Your body will digest it just like soda, meaning that it will go straight to your body cells and leave little for your brain cells. Fresh fruit breaks down slower and does a better job of satisfying your hunger. One hundred percent juice is still a better choice than soda—just be sure to keep your portions small (4 to 8 ounces per day).

? DID YOU KNOW?

Avocados are a fruit, but because of their high fat content, they are treated more like a fat. The fat in avocados is mostly monounsaturated and is very healthy for your brain.

Are you a sugar addict?

Unlike the natural sugar in fruit, foods with added sugars (specifically "sweets") actually trick your brain into overindulging in them, sort of like a drug. Think about the last time you were faced with a bowl of M&M's. Did you stop at just one? Or did you keep popping them into

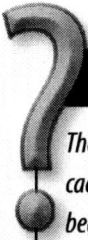

DID YOU KNOW?

The cacao ("kah-KAY-oh") bean is the base ingredient in chocolate. The percentage of cacao listed on a chocolate bar is the percentage that actually comes from the cacao bean. The higher the percentage of cacao, the more bitter the chocolate will taste.

your mouth until the bowl was all but empty? Now think about the last time you ate grapes. Chances are you didn't feel the same compulsion to eat more than a few handfuls. One reason it happens with M&M's is that they almost desensitize your taste buds to sugar, compelling you to eat more and more to taste the same level of sweetness you experienced in the first few bites.

Remember, it's okay to give your favorite sweet treats a place in your diet. Just make it a *small* place –your waistline will thank you. You'll also be pleasantly surprised to find that by limiting refined sugars, your taste buds adapt and you begin to prefer less sugary foods. A handful of grapes will probably cure your occasional "sweet tooth", and if not, eat a square of dark chocolate and be done with the craving.

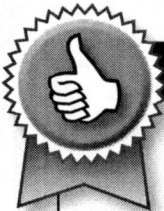

GOOD IDEA!

Hershey's Extra Dark Chocolate (60% cacao) is a delicious chocolate conveniently available in individually wrapped (binge-proof) one-square portion sizes. Each square is 45 calories, bittersweet and sure to tame even the most unrelenting sweet tooth!

Café Chocolate:

(45 calories)

1 square of Hershey's Extra Dark Chocolate (60% cacao)
6 oz. freshly brewed coffee

Place the square at the bottom of the coffee mug. Pour coffee over the chocolate and stir until melted.
Makes one serving.

FRUIT TOOTH POWER HABITS™!

✓ Stock your kitchen or dorm room with fresh fruit for when your sweet tooth attacks. Apples, bananas, pears, oranges and grapes are all very portable.

✓ If you can't get fresh fruit, fill your freezer with frozen fruit like strawberries, blueberries and peaches. If you don't have much freezer space, try unsweetened applesauce and dried fruit.

✓ For a snack, grab a cluster of grapes instead of a handful of M&M's.

✓ Top your morning bowl of oatmeal with sliced strawberries or a handful of raisins.

✓ When fruit just won't cut the craving and you must have candy, try a square of dark chocolate.

✓ Write your own Fruit Tooth Power Habit™: _____

_____

_____

The Bottom Line

Everyone has a "sweet tooth" that attacks once in a while. Get into the habit of eating fruit to cure yours and your taste buds will adapt. Start by picking some Fruit Tooth Power Habits™ from above or create your own to reduce the sugar in your diet and increase the fuel to your brain! Don't forget to record it on your Power Habit™ Tracking Chart in the back of the book!

Secret 8

VEG OUT!

What's in it for you?

✓ Give your skin a healthy glow

✓ Improve your concentration

✓ Stick to your healthy-eating goals once and for all

✓ Get and stay lean!

✓ Prevent two of the leading causes of death

✓ Develop a killer immune system

Recommendations:

✓ 2-3 cups of vegetables per day

If you're serious about wanting to look and feel better while keeping off the pounds, saying yes to vegetables is the first step

Your mom always said you should eat your vegetables and she was right for many reasons. Some of their benefits may surprise you.

? DID YOU KNOW?

Fresh vegetables aren't always the most nutritious. Once a vegetable is picked, it begins to lose nutritional value. Frozen vegetables are "flash-frozen" right after they're harvested, meaning they retain most of their nutrients.

What counts as a serving?

✓ 1 cup of raw or cooked vegetables

✓ 1 cup of vegetable juice

✓ 2 cups of raw leafy greens (arugula, cabbage, spinach, romaine lettuce, kale, mustard greens, collards)

✓ 1 cup of beans, legumes, corn, peas or potatoes

Two to three cups of vegetables might seem like a lot, but watch how fast it adds up each day:

Monday:

◇ Eat a side salad with your lunch: 1 cup

◇ Fill half your dinner plate with a hot vegetable such as steamed broccoli and carrots: 2 cups

Total: 3 cups of vegetables

Tuesday:

◇ Toss some mushrooms and onions into your morning omelet: half-cup

◇ Eat 14 baby carrots with peanut butter as a snack: 1 cup

◇ Order your pizza piled high with tomatoes, onion and green peppers: half-cup

Total: 2 cups of vegetables

Wednesday:

✧ Order (or make) a lunch smoothie made with 14 baby carrots: 1 cup

✧ Drink 8 ounces of low-sodium V8 juice for a snack: 1 cup

✧ Eat a medium baked potato with dinner: 1 cup

Total: 3 cups of vegetables

Thursday:

✧ Have a bowl of vegetable soup for lunch: ½ cup

✧ Order your Chipotle Burrito Bowl with extra fajita vegetables and black beans: 1½ cups

✧ Snack on a small bowl of cherry tomatoes: 1 cup

Total: 3 cups of vegetables

Friday:

✧ Eat a big salad for lunch: Fill a dinner plate with fresh spinach, chopped cucumbers, carrots, tomatoes, broccoli and celery; sprinkle with a little feta or shredded Cheddar cheese; and top with a few ounces of lean protein like grilled chicken or light tuna.

Total: 3 cups of vegetables (at least)

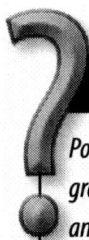

DID YOU KNOW?

Potatoes aren't fattening! One medium potato has 160 calories, 0 grams of fat, 4 grams of protein and 4 grams of fiber. That's hardly a high-calorie meal. How you top and prepare them can make them unhealthy. For example, a large order of french fries from McDonald's has 500 calories and 25 grams of fat. A "loaded" baked potato with butter, sour cream, bacon and cheese is packed with 480 calories and 29 grams of fat.

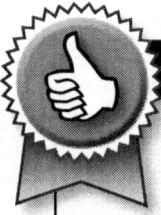

GOOD IDEA!

Always keep frozen vegetables in your freezer. If you can't squeeze them in during the day, you can always heat up a bowl in the evening.

Vegged-Out Tomato Soup:

(270 calories; 2 cups of vegetables)

1 can Amy's Organic Cream of Tomato Soup
1 cup frozen vegetable of your choice

Heat the soup in a microwave-safe bowl according to the instructions. Heat the vegetables in a microwave-safe bowl according to the instructions. Combine the soup and vegetables.
Makes one serving.

Your brain on veggies

Just like fruits, vegetables are high in antioxidants, which work to sweep up those damaging free radicals in your body. Because free radicals can have a negative effect on your brain function, you'll want to make sure veggies are on your plate at least twice a day. Vegetables with deeper and richer colors generally contain higher antioxidant levels.

Top-Scoring Antioxidant-Rich Veggies

(Source: USDA Database for the Oxygen Radical Absorbance Capacity (ORAC) of Selected Foods, May 2010)

✧ Artichokes
✧ Asparagus
✧ Beans and legumes
✧ Beets
✧ Bell Peppers
✧ Broccoli

✧ Cabbage
✧ Green leafy lettuce
✧ Onions
✧ Potatoes with skin (sweet and white)
✧ Radishes
✧ Spinach

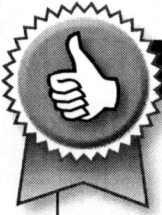

GOOD IDEA!

The next time you have spaghetti for dinner, instead of filling your plate with pasta and sauce, fill it with cooked vegetables (like spinach, peppers and broccoli), add about a cup of pasta and then add the marinara sauce. You'll cut down on the calories and boost your fiber. Bonus: For even more fiber, swap out the meatballs for a half-cup of beans or lentils.

The "domino effect" of veggies

Are you surrounded by so many tasty but unhealthy foods that you feel like you have to eat them? Certainly you can find salads and smoothies on campus, but the pizza and french fries (sorry, fries don't count as a vegetable) often overcrowd them. Let's face it, sometimes the less healthy option is just too tempting to pass up. Making a conscious effort to eat a serving or two of vegetables every day fixes this problem. Eating vegetables makes it easier to continue making better food choices. It creates a "domino effect" of good choices to follow and puts you in a better place mentally and physically. You just did something really good for your body, so you'll probably think twice before turning around and eating a greasy cheeseburger and fries at your next meal.

If you're serious about wanting to look and feel better while keeping off the pounds, saying yes to vegetables is the first step.

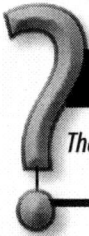

DID YOU KNOW?

Though they're prepared and served like vegetables, tomatoes are a fruit.

Get lean—eat your greens

Raw vegetables are low in fat and calories and high in fiber, take longer to chew and help you feel full. Starchy vegetables like potatoes, corn and peas are higher in calories. If you're thinking of eating a big plate of broccoli for dinner and expect to feel full, think again. By themselves, vegetables are too low in calories to keep you satisfied, so you'll need to pair them with other foods. Think about filling half your plate with non-starchy vegetables, a quarter with lean protein, a quarter with grain (or other carbohydrate-containing food such as starchy vegetables, fruit, milk or yogurt) and a little healthy fat to help it "stick."

Your Plate

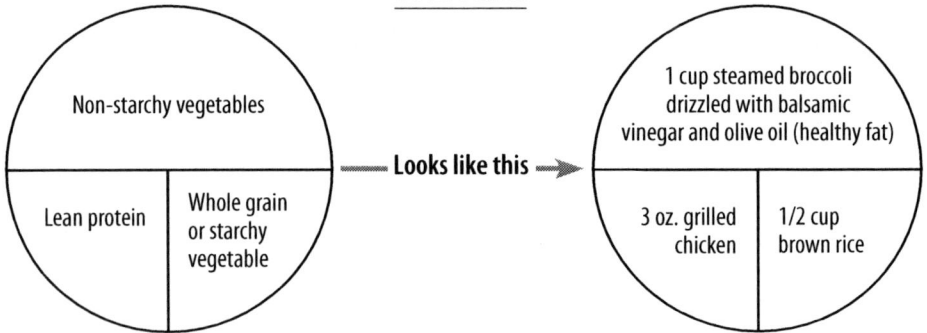

Non-starchy vegetables

Lean protein

Whole grain or starchy vegetable

Looks like this ➡

1 cup steamed broccoli drizzled with balsamic vinegar and olive oil (healthy fat)

3 oz. grilled chicken

1/2 cup brown rice

Your immune system on veggies

When your stress level is high due to the demands of classes, tests, papers or waiting for that hottie to text you back, you're more likely to catch a cold or come down with the flu. Eating vitamin C and beta-carotene-rich vegetables and fruits will help your body fight it because they strengthen your immune system. See Secret 7 for a list of fruits rich in vitamin C and beta-carotene.

Beta-Carotene-Rich Vegetables	Vitamin C-Rich Vegetables
Broccoli	Bell peppers
Carrots	Broccoli
Collard greens	Brussels sprouts
Kale	Green Cabbage
Romaine lettuce	Chile peppers
Spinach	Mustard greens
Sweet potatoes	Red cabbage
Turnip greens	Rutabagas
Winter squash	

Veggies: cheap health insurance

Fruits and vegetables are like health insurance you can buy at your local grocery store. According to the Centers for Disease Control and Prevention (CDC), compared with people who consume a diet with only small amounts of fruits and vegetables, those who eat more generous amounts reduce their risks of chronic diseases, cardiovascular diseases and cancer. The likelihood of having a stroke is also reduced. In most cases, cancer and heart disease are preventable, and eating your fruits and veggies is a small step you can take every day to protect yourself.

Your skin on veggies

Since your skin is the largest organ in your body, what you eat (or don't eat) will affect its health and appearance. Free radicals damage your skin cells and cause wrinkly looking skin. Antioxidants in fruits and vegetables remove these free radicals from your body, including your skin cells. You're young and vibrant, so your skin should be clear and smooth and have a healthy glow. When you're in your thirties and the cashier at the grocery store asks to see your driver's license before she scans your bottle of wine, you can thank the broccoli and apples you've been eating!

DID YOU KNOW?

Contrary to popular belief, fruits and vegetables aren't expensive. The price of a snack-size bag of potato chips is 93 cents, and the price of a medium apple is 70 cents.

VEG OUT POWER HABITS™!

✓ When you dine out, order a side of vegetables rather than a side of french fries.

✓ Make it a habit to fill a 3-cup food container with raw vegetables every day and snack on them when you get hungry. Baby carrots, sliced cucumbers, red pepper strips and cherry tomatoes all work great. If you need dip, try hummus.

✓ Most campus dining halls have a salad bar. Either have a salad with your meal or make it the main course by adding black beans and grilled chicken on top.

✓ When you make or order a smoothie, toss a handful of baby carrots or spinach into the blender along with skim milk and fruit. Not only does it make for a thicker consistency, but it also keeps you full for longer.

✓ Low-sodium V8 juice is a great snack you can carry in your bag. It comes in convenient 4-ounce cans and counts as a half-cup of vegetables.

✓ Write your own Veg Out Power Habit™: _____

_____

_____

The Bottom Line

Once you get into the habit of eating vegetables, you'll miss them if you skip a day. Pick some Veg Out Power Habits™ from the list above to practice today, or create your own. Even if you can't eat 2 to 3 cups every day, remember that some is better than none! Don't forget to record it on your Power Habit™ Tracking Chart in the back of the book!

Secret 9

ENERGIZE WITH H$_2$O

What's in it for you?

✓ Prevent constipation

✓ Feel energized

Recommendations:

✓ 6-12 cups of water every day

You need water to survive

Why water?

There's a good reason why water is the only liquid that will truly quench your thirst. Plain and simple, it does the best job of hydrating your body. And an added benefit is that it's calorie-free! You need water to survive. In fact, it makes up more than 50% of your body and about 85% of your brain.

One of the biggest bonuses of water is that it makes you feel alert. How many times have you felt fatigued and blamed it on school, lack of sleep or stress? They may be partly to blame, but dehydration can worsen the fatigue and stress brought on by college life. Dehydration happens when your body loses more fluid than it takes in. It can be caused by vomiting, diarrhea, excessive sweating, laxative use or simply not drinking enough fluid. Besides fatigue, signs of dehydration include:

✔ Headache

✔ Loss of appetite

✔ Flushed skin

✔ Heat intolerance

✔ Lightheadedness

✔ Dry mouth and eyes

✔ Dark urine with a strong odor

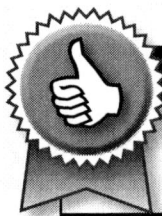

GOOD IDEA!

If you feel a headache coming on, don't reach for a pain reliever quite yet. Drink a cup of water—you might simply be dehydrated!

Besides making you feel energized, water benefits your body in the following ways:

✔ Regulates your body temperature

✔ Lubricates your joints

✔ Flushes out waste products

✔ Carries nutrients and oxygen to your cells

✔ Prevents and alleviates constipation

✔ Helps dissolve nutrients from the food you eat so that your body can use them

How much should *you* drink?

Water recommendations are based on several factors:

✓ How physically active you are

✓ How much you weigh

✓ How hot it is outside

✓ If you're sick with a fever and are vomiting or have diarrhea

✓ How thirsty you are

Keep in mind that once you begin feeling thirsty, your body is already dehydrated, so don't wait until you get to that point.

The general guideline is to drink from 6 to 12 cups of water a day. A quick way to determine your estimated water needs is to divide your body weight in pounds by 2. The result is the approximate number of ounces of water you need every day, not taking into account exercise or illness. For example, if you weigh 175 pounds, you need about 88 ounces of water a day, or about five or six tall (16-ounce) glasses.

The best way to check how hydrated you are is to check the color of your urine. Really! If it's a pale yellow color, you're pretty well hydrated. If it looks like the color of apple juice or beer, you'd better drink up!

DID YOU KNOW?

Bottled waters are typically not better for you than plain old tap water. Bottled waters lack fluoride, an essential mineral for strong teeth. Tap water has all the fluoride you need!

What else can you drink?

Water comes in many forms, and they all count toward your daily fluid requirements. They aren't all created equal, though. Consider these beverages:

1. Gatorade and other sports drinks

Gatorade was created as a beverage to help the Florida Gators football team perform better during practice and games. As they sweat, they lost important electrolytes responsible for the body's chemical balance (specifically sodium, potassium and chloride). As a result, they weren't playing as well as they could have been.

Scientists formulated a beverage to replenish these electrolytes, and Gatorade was born. It was created for athletes, but today it's consumed by athletes and non-athletes alike. The problem is, if you're drinking Gatorade to meet your fluid needs but aren't participating in prolonged physical activity and sweating a lot, you'll be taking in a bunch of extra calories that you probably won't burn off. In this case, water is the better choice for you.

A 32-ounce bottle of Gatorade has 200 calories, 440 mg of sodium and 56 grams of sugar. If you drink two bottles of Gatorade every day, that's 400 extra calories and 880 milligrams of sodium per day.

Again, Gatorade is a perfectly suitable choice if you're participating in vigorous physical activity, but not when you're sitting at your desk for hours on end.

DID YOU KNOW?

Coconut water is the liquid found inside young green coconuts. It's different from coconut milk in that it's fat-free and much lower in calories and contains sodium, magnesium, potassium, chloride and calcium—all essential electrolytes. For this reason, coconut water is a fantastic natural sports drink! The three most popular brands you'll find at the grocery store are Zico, Vita Coco and O.N.E. Because coconut water has sodium (160 mg per 14-ounce bottle of Zico coconut water), you shouldn't drink it like water. Your best bet is to enjoy a bottle after a rigorous, sweaty workout.

2. Coffee, tea and other caffeinated beverages

Although once thought to dehydrate your body, scientists have determined that there's no truth behind the caffeine-dehydration argument as long as you drink it in moderation. Drinking a cup of coffee in the morning to get you going counts, but don't forget to count the extra calories from the cream and sugar. For example, a grande Caffé Mocha with whipped cream from Starbucks has a whopping 330 calories, 15 grams of fat, 8 grams of saturated fat and 33 grams of sugar!

If you're a healthy college student, moderate amounts of caffeine (200 to 300 mg per day—one to two cups of coffee depending on strength) usually don't cause problems. When you overdo it, caffeine can give you the jitters and interfere with your sleep. If you're caffeine-sensitive, you could experience this nervousness with just one cup.

DID YOU KNOW?

When it comes to soft drinks, Vault has the most caffeine (71 mg) per 12-ounce serving, followed by diet and regular Mountain Dew (54 mg) and then Diet Coke (47 mg).

The caffeine content of your favorite drinks:

- ✧ Coffee (8 oz.): 95-200 mg
- ✧ Black tea (8 oz.): 40-120 mg
- ✧ Green tea (6 oz.): 26 mg
- ✧ Iced tea (12-16 oz.): 7-27 mg
- ✧ Espresso (1 oz.): 58-75 mg
- ✧ Energy drinks (8 oz.): 74-280 mg
- ✧ Soft drinks: (12 oz.): 23-71 mg

DID YOU KNOW?

In moderation, caffeine can boost your brain function, making you more alert.

Since I can't have caffeine, to survive my 8:00 a.m. classes I would eat a role of Sweet Tarts during class to stay awake. By the end of college, I had four cavities!

— TAMMY, graduate of Shawnee State University

3. Soft drinks and diet soft drinks

Yes, they both count toward your fluid needs, but you want to go easy on them. Just like sports drinks and sweetened coffee drinks, regular soft drinks pack a sugary, calorie-loaded punch. Sugary beverages also cause the crash-and-burn effect. They give you immediate energy in the form of simple carbohydrates, which means you digest them rapidly and then crash and burn.

Diet soft drinks contain artificial sweeteners and can actually make you crave sugar because they're so much sweeter than regular table sugar.

4. Alcohol

Beer, wine and hard liquor dehydrate your body and don't count toward your water needs. Actually, they have the opposite effect. Alcohol triggers your kidneys to produce more urine. The more you urinate, the more dehydrated you become.

5. Flavored water and vitamin-enhanced water:

Some flavored waters are sweetened with real juice, others with artificial sweeteners. Read the label and go for the natural sweeteners. Artificial sweeteners include:

✓ Acesulfame potassium (Sunett, Sweet One)

✓ Aspartame (Equal, NutraSweet)

✓ Neotame

✓ Saccharin (SugarTwin, Sweet'N Low)

✓ Sucralose (Splenda)

Vitamin water can be a nice change of pace from regular water once in a while but should never replace pure water. They can get pretty expensive, too! Drinking one bottle of vitamin-enhanced water a day will add up to about $400 by the end of the year! See the table below for more information on some of the many waters on the market today.

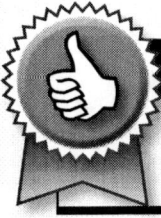

GOOD IDEA!

Make your own flavored water. Add a tablespoon of your favorite 100% fruit juice to 16 ounces of water. Calories: 10

Flavored water:	How's it flavored?	Calories per serving
Hint	Infused with natural flavors	0
SoBe Lifewater	Sugar, natural flavors	100
SoBe Zero Calorie Lifewater	Reb A (purified Stevia extract), erythritol*	0
Glaceau Vitamin Water	Crystalline fructose, natural flavor	125
Glaceau Vitamin Water Zero	Rebiana (Stevia extract), Crystalline fructose and erythritol*	0
Propel Fitness Water	Sucrose syrup, natural flavors, **sucralose****	30
Aquafina FlavorSplash	Natural flavors, **sucralose****	0
Dasani Flavored Water	Natural flavor, **sucralose****	0
Clearly Canadian Sparkling Water	Cane sugar, natural flavor, **sucralose****	45 per 8 oz.

*Sugar alcohol **Artificial sweetener

6. ***Bottled water:***

Bottled water is a fine choice—just be sure it has fluoride. The following bottled-water companies carry fluoridated options:

✓ Arrowhead
✓ Deer Park
✓ Ice Mountain
✓ Poland Springs
✓ Zephyrhills

H$_2$O POWER HABITS™!

✓ Replace that 12-ounce can of soda with 12 ounces of water.

✓ Make it a habit to carry a water bottle with you to class and sip on it throughout the day.

✓ If you like your water with a little flavor, drop in a cucumber slice or squeeze a few drops of lemon, lime or orange juice into it. True Lemon makes small packets of crystallized lemon, lime and orange to mix into your water for flavor without the calories or artificial sweeteners.

✓ If you choose a fruit drink or other sugary beverage, dilute it with water.

✓ Drink 8 ounces of water between each of your meals.

✓ Drink 8 ounces of water with each of your meals.

✓ Write your own H$_2$O Power Habit™: _____

_____

_____

The Bottom Line

Find your water balance by checking the color of your urine. Drink a little more water if it's the color of beer. Choose from the H$_2$O Power Habits™ above and get energized! Don't forget to record it on your Power Habit™ Tracking Chart in the back of the book!

Secret 10

GO WITH YOUR GUT

What's in it for you?

✓ Stop eating your way through stress

✓ Put an end to overeating

✓ Lose weight without counting calories

Treat your fork like a fork, not a shovel.

Why not stuff your face?

You need a certain number of calories to maintain your current weight. When you eat too much on a regular basis and you don't burn off enough of those calories with exercise, you store the extra calories as fat and the number on your bathroom scale goes up.

Overeating causes your digestive system to work overtime, too. Think about Thanksgiving dinner. Don't you feel like taking a nap after you shovel in the traditional feast? You may blame it on the turkey, but it's actually the extra calories you just ate. You've just given your body a huge job to do, so now your blood is forced to travel to your digestive system to start processing all that food. You feel sluggish after a large meal because your body is undergoing an extreme digestive workout. To avoid slipping into a food coma, eat less.

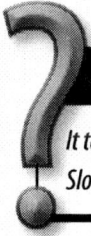

DID YOU KNOW?

It takes about 20 minutes for your brain to recognize that you've had enough to eat. Slow down!

How can you tell if you're overeating?

If you've been an overeater for most of your life, you may not even realize you're doing it. Or you might be in denial but your tight-fitting jeans are telling a different story. If this is you, don't worry—you can fix it. You just have to have a little patience and get to know your stomach a little better.

DID YOU KNOW?

Your stomach can stretch to hold as much as 128 ounces (the size of a gallon of milk). Its natural capacity, however, is 32 ounces (the size of a large bottle of Gatorade).

Think of food like fuel for your car. You depend on it for energy just like your car depends on gas to move. When you "top off" your gas tank, your car doesn't go faster or function any better than if you filled it halfway. And not only will topping off your stomach not help you to go further, but it will slow you down and make you feel sleepy.

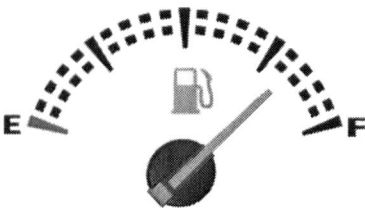

Picture your stomach with a gauge connected to it that moves from "empty" to "full" as you feed it. Better yet, pretend it goes from 0 to 5. See the scale below to help you visualize this concept:

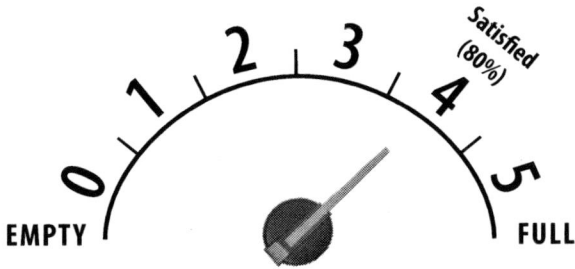

Level "0" or "empty"

At "0," you're empty and coasting on fumes. Your stomach is the size of your fist. You're famished and you don't have any mental or physical energy. Read a chapter for class? Forget it. You can't even focus on the television. You need food fast, and because your eyes are bigger than your stomach when you're in this state, once you start eating you'll probably eat too much.

Level "4" or "80%"

You don't feel hungry but you also don't feel full. Level 4 is considered "satisfied". Most people eat beyond that level and don't realize it. Physical energy and mental focus are at their peak here, so it's important to understand what this feels like and strive for it. You'll learn more about this in a moment.

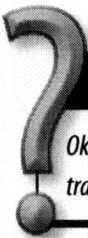

DID YOU KNOW?

Okinawans practice calorie control with a habit called "hara hachi bu," which translates into "eat until you're 80% full". Level 4 is considered 80% full.

Level "5" or "full"

Your stomach is filled to its natural capacity (32 ounces). You aren't stuffed yet, but you've definitely had enough to eat.

Levels 6-10 (the Overeating Zone)

You're more than full and your stomach is stretching to accommodate all the food that's in it. Many people overeat simply because it's what they're used to doing. Rather than using a gas gauge that ranges from 0 to 5, they use one that extends to 10. There's more than one level in the overeating range, as you'll see on the scale below.

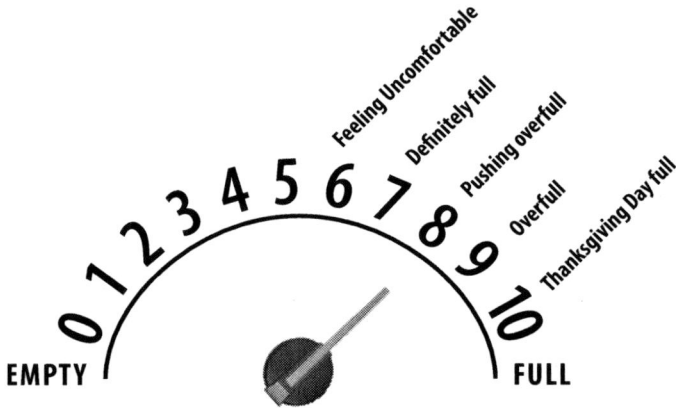

At the most extreme end of the zone (level 10), you're topped off and couldn't eat another bite if someone paid you. Your stomach is about the size of a gallon of milk (really!). Another way to describe level 10 is "Thanksgiving Day-full." You can't even keep your eyes open, let alone read a chapter for class.

Now back to level "4." There are two reasons why it's so important to know what this level feels like:

1. *It will help keep you from packing on those dreadful college pounds. When you identify your "4" and strive to eat closer to it at meals, you'll be eating less (though enough to fuel your body).*

2. *You'll have more energy left to spend time with your friends, exercise and study.*

So, how do you go from eating to a level 6, 7, 8, 9 or 10 to eating to a level 4? The first step is to redefine your scale. Instead of a 0-10 scale, your new scale should stop at 5. This doesn't mean you'll never eat past a level 5 again, but that won't be the norm.

The second step is to "connect" with your stomach and get to know it a little better. Believe it or not, you used to be a "connected" eater. You were born with a finely tuned sense of hunger and fullness. If you don't believe it, the next time you have the opportunity, watch a baby as she's being bottle-fed. She stops when she feels satisfied, drinking not an ounce more. Even if Mom tries to force that extra ounce, she won't drink it. She turns her head, and if Mom persists, she'll push the bottle away because she's at her "4." She instinctively knows not to eat any more.

Give yourself permission to eat like a baby.

Where did this "connection" go? What happened? More important, how can you get it back and enjoy a healthier weight, more energy and a supercharged brain?

In a word, life is what happened. Maybe your parents made you clean your plate growing up and you got used to always feeling stuffed. This level became your "4", so you really don't feel like you're overeating. But the truth is, if you clean your plate at every meal, you're probably overeating.

Maybe you use food to cope with life. Do you ever find yourself eating when you aren't hungry? Maybe you eat when you're bored, stressed, sad, angry, anxious, depressed or happy. We all do this to some degree— it's called "head hunger." Eating for emotional reasons is a sure sign of a "disconnect," because you're feeding your stomach when it isn't hungry. When was the last time you saw a baby cry because he needed a diaper change and Mom came running with a bottle? She tried to feed him, but he kept crying. If he could have talked, he might have said: "Hey, dummy, check the diaper! I'm wet and uncomfortable. I don't want to eat!" He's upset but doesn't turn to food to ease his emotions, because he knows it won't work.

Feeding your head hunger is a learned response. You can unlearn it.

GOOD IDEA!

If you have a candy dish or other container full of candy in your dorm or apartment, get rid of it. Otherwise, you may end up seeking comfort in it when you're stressed.

It's really not difficult to become a more connected eater. All you have to do is follow the seven simple steps below and you're on your way. Keep in mind that you didn't become an overeater overnight, so don't expect to break the habit overnight. It takes about 21 days to build or break an eating habit, so keep practicing these steps until they feel normal, and whatever you do, don't give up on yourself!

7 steps to connecting with your stomach

Step 1: Think of your stomach as a 32-ounce container

The natural capacity of your stomach is 32 ounces (about 4 cups)

Step 2: Get hydrated

Your body interprets dehydration as hunger. Drink 8 to 16 ounces of water before a meal just to be sure.

Step 3: Find your hara hachi bu (level 4)

How much food does it take for you to feel satisfied? The amount depends on what you're eating and will be different for everyone. If you know what "0" feels like, start from there and slowly "add food." Once you hit "4" (satisfied), stop eating and wait. Because it takes about 20 minutes for your brain to recognize that you're satisfied, if you stop at a level 4, twenty minutes later you'll be at a level 5.

Step 4: Slow down!

The faster you eat, the more you eat. Before you know it, you're at a level 7 or 8.

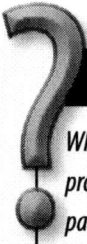

DID YOU KNOW?

When you drink your calories rather than chew them, you won't feel as satisfied and probably won't cut calories elsewhere in your diet to compensate. Wonder why your pants won't zip?

Step 5: Just eat!

How many times have you found yourself eating while watching television, checking your friends' Facebook posts, reading or working on a project? It's too easy to become disconnected when you're involved in other activities while eating. During meals, pick a place to eat, like your kitchen table, a dining-hall table or your desk, and do only that—eat! Facebook can wait 15 minutes.

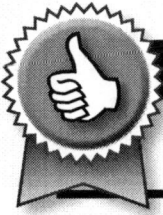

GOOD IDEA!

Never, never, never eat straight from the bag unless it's a bag of carrots!

Step 6: Mind your portions

When you know what a real portion size looks like, you're one step closer to controlling how much you eat. The old saying "Your eyes are bigger than your stomach" is often true. We load our plates mindlessly with large portions of food when we're hungry without giving it a second thought, but if it's not on your plate, you won't eat it. It doesn't help that portion sizes have exploded over the past 20 years. Take a look at the following examples and see if you're convinced:

20 years ago	Today
Bagel = 120 calories	Bagel = 350 calories
Fast-food hamburger = 333 calories	Fast-food hamburger = 590 calories
Spaghetti and meatballs = 500 calories	Spaghetti and meatballs = 1,025 calories

20 years ago	Today
Soda (6.5 oz.) = 85 calories	Soda (20-oz. portion) = 250 calories
French fries (2.4 oz.) = 210 calories	French fries (6.9 oz.) = 610 calories
Turkey sandwich = 320 calories	Turkey sandwich = 820 calories
8-oz. coffee with milk and sugar = 45 calories	Venti Caffè Mocha with whipped cream = 410 calories
Blueberry muffin (1.5 oz.) = 210 calories	Blueberry muffin (5 oz.) = 500 calories
2 slices of pepperoni pizza = 500 calories	2 large slices of pepperoni pizza = 850 calories
Box of movie popcorn = 270 calories	Tub of movie popcorn = 630 calories
Cheesecake (3 oz.) = 260 calories	Cheesecake = 640 calories
Chocolate-chip cookie = 55 calories	Chocolate chip cookie = 275 calories
Chicken stir-fry = 435 calories	Chicken stir-fry = 865 calories

Source: Department of Health and Human Services http://hp2010.nhlbihin.net/portion/

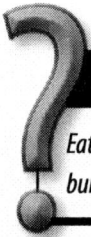

DID YOU KNOW?

Eating late at night won't cause you to gain weight. Eating more calories than you burn is what puts on the pounds, not the time of day.

GOOD IDEA!

Use salad plates instead of dinner plates at meal times—you'll eat less that way, but it won't feel like it!

Now take a look at what a portion is supposed to look like:

Common portion equivalent	Serving size	Equals 1 portion of
Truffle	1 tablespoon	Peanut butter
Baseball	1 cup	-Fruit or vegetables -Cereal (flakes or rounds)
Golf ball	2 tablespoons	Hummus
Computer mouse	1 each	Size of a medium potato
Deck of cards or an iPhone	3 oz.	Beef or chicken
Checkbook	3 oz.	Fish
Stamp	1 teaspoon	Oil
Tennis ball	½ cup	-Beans or potatoes -Hot cereal -Cooked pasta or rice -Dried fruit
6 stacked dice	1½ oz.	Cheese
Egg	¼ cup	-Granola -Beans (1 oz. meat)
CD	1 each	Pancake or waffle
Yo-yo	1 oz.	Dinner roll
Hockey puck	1 oz.	½ medium bagel

Step 7: *Find out what's eating you*

To figure out what's prompting you to eat when you're not hungry, keep a weeklong food journal in which you take the following steps (a sample journal is shown below as well as in the appendix):

   a. Write down everything you eat and drink.

   b. Assign a number to your hunger/fullness before and after you eat.

c. Do you see a pattern where you're eating even though you aren't hungry? Identify the reason and write it down. Did something happen, causing you to turn to food for comfort? Did you do poorly on an exam? Did your boyfriend or girlfriend just dump you? Are you stressed out about something? Are you procrastinating rather than writing that paper? Are you sad or lonely? You may be surprised to discover the number of times you reach for a snack for reasons like these.

d. Once you identify the source, it's time to cope. Find another outlet. Sit with your feelings and really experience them.

e. You may still find yourself turning toward food for comfort even after Step D. That's okay. It's what you're used to, so it's going to take some time to break this old habit. Try developing new coping skills. For example, if you eat when you're stressed, stop and do 10 jumping jacks or push-ups. Nothing tackles stress better than exercise. It doesn't have to be a full workout. Think quick and effective. The more you practice your new coping skills, the more automatic they'll become.

Expect to be stressed as a college student. In Secret 15, you'll learn some tips on how to best manage it, including stress-busting foods to eat for meals and snacks.

Food will never solve what's really bugging you—ever!

Eating to feed your head hunger is tough on your body and brain. It's an energy-draining habit because you never really get to the root of the problem. Food will never solve what's really bugging you—ever!

Food Journal

Hunger or fullness level before I ate (1-10)	What did I eat? What did I drink?	Hunger or fullness level when I stopped eating (1-10)	How am I feeling? Sad, happy, depressed, angry, lonely, stressed, etc.	If I'm feeding my "head hunger", how can I cope next time?
5	A big bowl of potato chips and a few handfuls of M&M's	8	Stressed out! This is finals week!	I'll get up and take a break and maybe do a few jumping jacks or push-ups.

GO WITH YOUR GUT POWER HABITS™!

✓ Redefine your gas tank. Use the 1-5 scale instead of 1-10.

✓ Be mindful when you eat today. Assign a number to your hunger and fullness and get to know your level "4."

✓ Slow down! Savor each bite. Remember, the faster you eat, the more you eat.

✓ Drink 8 to 16 ounces of water before a meal and before you reach for a snack. You may actually be thirsty or dehydrated, not hungry.

✓ During meals, pick a place to eat, like your kitchen table, a dining-hall table or at your desk, and do only that—eat!

✓ Mind your portions. Match your portion sizes with common objects (see chart) to be sure you aren't overeating.

✓ If you find yourself eating when you aren't hungry, find out why and develop a new coping skill. Put the skill to use every time you reach for food to feed your head hunger.

✓ Write your own Go With Your Gut Power Habit™: _____

_____

_____

The Bottom Line

Overeating is hard on your body. Get a handle on it, but be patient. Don't beat yourself up if you slip up. Get started by picking the Go With Your Gut Power Habit™ you're most comfortable with and practice it today. Don't forget to record it on your Power Habit™ Tracking Chart in the back of the book!

Secret 11

MOVE YOUR BUTT!

What's in it for you?

✓ Have hours of energy

✓ Burn more calories

✓ Feel happy

✓ Tackle your stress

Recommendations:

✓ 30 minutes of physical activity most days of the week

(Exercise minutes don't have to be consecutive.
They can be spread throughout the day.)

As a college student, you know that exercise is important. Not only does it burn off those extra calories from pizza, fries, burgers and beer, but it keeps the most important muscle in your body in shape—your heart. Something you probably haven't considered is how exercise gives you hours of extra energy and helps you stay focused. No, that's not what energy drinks and Caffé Mochas are for! Sure, caffeine gives you a jolt of immediate energy, but it doesn't last the entire day. In fact, because of the high sugar content of some of these beverages, you'll experience a crash-and-burn effect once the caffeine wears off. Not exactly what you bargained for.

DID YOU KNOW?

Energy drinks have 9.75 teaspoons of sugar per 12-ounce can!

The summer before college, I heard a lot about the notorious "freshman 15." I went to school with a goal to avoid it by eating healthy and working out a ton at the campus gym during the week. This would help counterbalance the weekend partying and the late-night appetite that comes with it (especially when you're walking back to the dorm and pass places to chow down like Raising Canes Chicken Fingers and Five Guys Burgers).

—NICK, sophomore at Ohio State University

DID YOU KNOW?

One pound of body fat equals 3,500 calories. To lose 1 pound, you have to burn 3,500 calories over the course of a week by eating a little less or exercising a little more or both. This means that if you pig out and party over the weekend, it's going to take more than 30 minutes on the treadmill to undo the damage.

Calories Burned in 1 Hour

(For a 160-pound person)

Activity:	Calories burned:	Like burning off:
Aerobics, high impact	511	Large bagel with cream cheese
Aerobics, low impact	365	Starbucks' chocolate chunk cookie
Aerobics, water	292	Beer (two 12-oz. bottles)
Basketball game	584	Pepperoni pizza (2 slices)
Bicycling, <10mph	292	Ham and cheese omelet
Football, touch, flag, general	584	Chocolate milkshake (12 oz.)
Hiking	438	McDonald's double cheeseburger
Ice skating	511	Spaghetti with meat sauce (lunch-size portion)
Jogging, 5 mph	584	Subway 6" chicken and bacon ranch sub
Racquetball, casual	511	Chicken Caesar salad with dressing
Rollerblading	913	Bag of Butter Lover's microwave popcorn, 20-oz Coke, 6 Twizzlers
Rope jumping	730	Stack of pancakes with syrup
Rowing, stationary	511	Large order of french fries
Running, 8 mph	986	Chipotle chicken fajita burrito
Skiing, cross-country	511	Loaded baked potato
Skiing, downhill	365	Container of ramen noodle soup
Softball or baseball	365	Hot dog in a bun with ketchup and mustard
Swimming, laps	511	Venti white-chocolate mocha
Tae kwon do	730	10 chicken wings with sauce
Tai chi	292	Macaroni and cheese (1 serving)
Tennis, singles	584	Hot fudge sundae
Volleyball	292	Potato chips (2 oz.)
Walking, 3.5 mph	277	Breakfast sausage (3 links)
Weightlifting, free weight, Nautilus or universal type	219	Chocolate cake with frosting (1 slice)

Source: Mayo Clinic website http://www.mayoclinic.com/health/exercise/SM00109

Exercise and energize your body

When you're sitting in class or at your desk studying, your body is at rest. The blood vessels in your muscles are working like a garden hose, with a nice steady blood flow. When you exercise those same muscles with a brisk walk, jog or stair-climbing session, those same blood vessels work like fire hoses—all-out maximum-force blood flow! Afterward, you can feel little energizing twitches in your legs and arms, which is why it's so difficult to fall asleep after a jog. Your body doesn't want to sleep—it's too pumped up! Your blood is responsible for delivering oxygen and nutrients to all the cells of your body. When your blood flows like a fire hose, more oxygen and nutrients get carried to those cells, contributing to that energized feeling.

No amount of energy drink can compete with the lasting energy produced by exercise. The best news is that this energy stretches for hours past the time you stopped exercising. This means that if you exercise first thing in the morning, you'll feel awake and energized all the way through lunch!

I find it very helpful to take advantage of the rec center for at least an hour every day to stay healthy.

—NICOLE, sophomore at Ashland University

DID YOU KNOW?

Some experts say the best time of day to exercise is first thing in the morning, while others say late afternoon. I say the best time to exercise is when you're most likely to do it. Pick a time that works for you and just do it!

DID YOU KNOW?

Research by the American College of Sports Medicine shows that college students who participate in vigorous exercise get better grades than those who don't.

Exercise and energize your brain

Your brain loves exercise. The increase in heart rate that comes with exercise means your brain is literally being nourished with oxygenated blood. Studies have shown that exercise plays an important role in memory and learning. It improves blood flow to your brain and grows new brain cells. Just imagine how this can improve your grades!

Exercise is the most effective remedy for the "brain fuzzies," too. You know what those are—you sit down and try to work on a project and you can't seem to focus. Your mind is everywhere but where it needs to be, and you find yourself staring off into space. The best thing for you to do is get up and take a brisk five-minute walk to get the blood flowing back to your brain like the water surging through a fire hose.

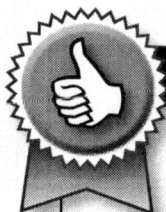

GOOD IDEA!

Set yourself up to work out. Schedule it on your calendar like a doctor's appointment and lay your exercise clothes on your bed where you can see them. That way, when you come home from class, all you have to do is get dressed and work out. No excuses!

Exercise and beat your stress

How often do you turn to food to cope with your stress? A handful of Hershey's Kisses here or a bag of potato chips there will never reduce your stress level or lower your anxiety. All these empty calories will do is steal your energy and make you gain weight.

A little stress can be a good thing, but there's no better way to beat the extra stresses of college than with exercise. Twenty minutes on the stair climber or elliptical machine releases feel-good chemicals called endorphins. They change your body's response to stress and give you a better outlook on life. Suddenly, things don't seem so bad. Endorphins are what give runners "runner's high," but they can also be felt with other forms of physical activity, too. Take your pick!

I didn't do much in the way of exercise until I was in my last year of college. Had I realized sooner how much it helped me cope with stress, I would have started exercising the day I moved into the dorms!

—ALAN, graduate of the University of Arizona

Exercise and beat the blues

One thing is for sure—you will never feel worse after you exercise.

Maybe you're homesick or lonely. Maybe you're struggling to find out where you fit in. Are you so uncertain about what to major in that you're wondering if you even belong in college? Each of these situations can cause mild to moderate depression and anxiety. Exercise is probably the last thing you want to do when you're feeling blue, but it will help you feel better and give you a more positive outlook. Did you know that inactive people are twice as likely to experience mild to moderate depression as people who are more active? You can thank those exercise endorphins for that. The bottom line is that exercise makes you feel good and boosts your self-esteem. One thing is for sure—you'll never feel worse after you exercise.

If you're feeling depressed or overwhelmed and it doesn't seem to be getting any better, seek help by visiting your campus counseling center. Remember, even when you feel like you're all alone, there are people who care about you and want to help you.

Exercise and beat the flu

Proper nutrition is important for a killer immune system, but exercise has the power to make your immune system even stronger. You don't have to jog five miles a day to protect your immune system. In fact, as little as 20 minutes of brisk walking five days a week is enough to do the trick. Count the number of minutes you spend walking swiftly to and from class each day and you might be surprised by how fast the minutes add up.

Dorm-room workouts

Good news! You can get an awesome workout without even leaving your dorm or apartment. Here's a list of some great inexpensive workout DVDs available online at amazon.com and collagevideo.com.

Workout DVD	Level
Crunch—Burn & Firm Pilates	Beginner/intermediate
Fat-Burning Kickboxing for Dummies	Beginner/intermediate
The Firm: Power Yoga	Beginner/intermediate
Walk Away the Pounds, by Leslie Sansone	Beginner/intermediate
10 Minute Solution: Rapid Results Pilates	Intermediate
Dance Off the Inches: Fat Burning Jam, by Michelle Dozois	Intermediate
Jackie Warner's Xtreme Timesaver Training	Intermediate
The Biggest Loser Workout: Cardio Max	Intermediate
The Biggest Loser Workout: Power Sculpt	Intermediate
The Firm: Total Body Makeover	Intermediate
Tight on Time: Hot Spots with Tamilee Webb	Intermediate
Build Up Your Muscles, by Gin Miller	Intermediate/advanced
Get Ripped: Slim & Lean with Jari Love	Advanced
Jillian Michaels' 30 Day Shred	Advanced
Patrick Goudeau Step Up	Advanced
1 Minute Workout: Total Body Toning, by Minna Lessig	You pick the level of intensity

I'm often asked by college students, "What's the best exercise to help me lose weight?" My reply is always the same: The one you will do and do consistently.

Lose the excuses

Unless you find a type of exercise you truly enjoy, you can always find something that sounds more appealing and talk yourself out of your workout. If you find yourself checking the Facebook statuses of your 855 "friends" or watching reruns of old sitcoms when you're supposed to be at the gym, you should probably find some more rewarding forms of exercise. That said, this is also where your accountability comes into play. Self-accountability is what drives you to step onto the treadmill when all you really feeling like doing is watching TV. The best exercise is the one you'll do. You don't have to run marathons. Think simple. The bottom line is that no one can make you exercise. You have to want to do it, commit to doing it and then just do it!

BUTT-MOVIN' POWER HABITS™!

✓ Schedule exercise time on your calendar like you do your classes and commit.

✓ Take the stairs instead of the elevator at every opportunity. If you live on the fourth floor of your residence hall or apartment, think of how many calories you'll burn if you take the stairs every day. Remember, the 30-minutes-a-day exercise recommendation can be spread out. Five minutes here and there all count toward the total!

✓ Find an exercise buddy and work out with him or her at scheduled times each week. You'll be much less likely to skip when your friend is counting on you.

✓ Lace up your tennis shoes and walk! Walking to class counts if you're doing it briskly enough to raise your heart rate.

✓ Take advantage of your campus recreation center. Whether you prefer swimming, group exercise classes, the treadmill or the elliptical machine, your campus fitness center is one of the true gems at your university. If you don't know how to work a piece of exercise equipment, ask a fitness-center staff person.

✓ Write your own Butt-Movin' Power Habit™: _____

_____

_____

The Bottom Line

Unwrap all your excuses for not exercising. Are they really the barriers you make them out to be? Do something, anything! Start with five minutes of exercise and build on it. Pick a Butt-Movin' Power Habit™ to commit to and get movin'! Don't forget to record it on your Power Habit™ Tracking Chart in the back of the book!

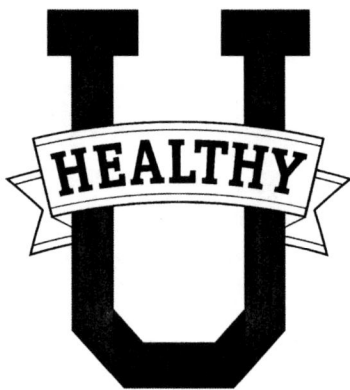

Secret 12

DRINK SMART

If you party and drink alcohol, be safe and smart and you'll avoid:

✓ A beer belly

✓ Sleepless nights

✓ Physical and mental energy drain

✓ Getting sick and feeling run down

✓ Poor skin health

Alcohol turns on your appetite "switch"

Your six-pack on a six-pack:

Just like overeating, overdrinking forces your body to pack on pounds of fat. Alcohol contains 7 calories per gram, almost as much as fat. The difference is that alcohol supplies "empty calories," or calories without nutrition. Because you're drinking the calories instead of eating them, you tend not to "count" them, but boy do they count! Some beverages contain as many calories as an entire meal. Check it out:

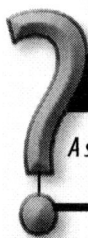

DID YOU KNOW?

A six-pack of beer has the same amount of calories as 12 chicken wings in sauce.

Drinking this much alcohol	Has this many calories	It's like eating
12 oz. of beer	145	2 chicken wings
A 6-pack of beer	870	12 chicken wings
12 oz. of light beer	110	3 cups Butter Lover's Popcorn
A 6-pack of light beer	660	2 slices of pizza
5 oz. of red wine	105	1 tablespoon of peanut butter
5 oz. of white wine	100	1 tablespoon of peanut butter
12-oz. margarita	550	2 Ham & Cheese Hot Pockets
Chocolate martini	435	1 peanut butter and jelly sandwich
Apple Martini	235	1 packet of Easy Mac-n-Cheese
12-oz. Mudslide	839	Half-bag of potato chips
Mixed Drinks		
Whiskey sour	125	1 scoop of ice cream
Energy drink & vodka	180	1 serving of ramen noodles
Rum & Coke	170	1 chocolate brownie
Cosmopolitan	215	Half a peanut butter and jelly sandwich
Daiquiri	250	Small cherry sundae
1 Shot of Hard Liquor		
Vodka		
Rum	100	2 small chocolate chip cookies
Gin		
Tequila		

DID YOU KNOW?

A 12-ounce bottle of beer has the same amount of liquor as 1 shot of 80-proof liquor or 5 ounces of wine. Drinking six beers is like drinking six glasses of wine or doing six shots. Ouch!

It doesn't take much alcohol to pack on the pounds. Let's say you drink six bottles of light beer over the course of the weekend (660 calories). If you get into the habit of doing this every weekend and don't burn off the calories or subtract them elsewhere in your diet, in five weeks you'll be 1 pound heavier—and that's if you drink light beer. That's also not factoring in the pizza or the Taco Bell order you're wolfing down after a long night of partying. That 1 pound can very quickly turn into 2 pounds, and by the end of the school year you'll be 10 to 15 pounds heavier. So much for that spring-break bikini body or the six-pack abs you were hoping for! Think before you drink.

Appetite, meet alcohol

Alcohol turns on your appetite "switch." It's as if a little voice in your head whispers: "Go ahead, eat it. It doesn't count." So not only are you taking in the calories from alcohol, but you're also filling your body with extra food calories. Face it, you're not reaching for carrot sticks and apple slices when you're drinking. It's more like chips, burgers, french fries and pizza.

DID YOU KNOW?

24 beers = 1 pound of body fat. And 19 Red Bull & vodkas = 1 pound of body fat.

Alcohol and the morning after

When you have one too many drinks, your physical and mental energy are zapped the next day. In addition to the physical symptoms of a hangover (headache, dry mouth, unsettled stomach), your body's ability to absorb several vitamins and minerals is also diminished. Why should you care? These are the same vitamins and minerals that help get you through the day with energy and laser focus. Other typical side effects of drinking too much alcohol include:

- ✓ Fatigue
- ✓ Irritability
- ✓ Insomnia
- ✓ Poor skin health

If you're going to drink, set a limit and ask a friend to hold you accountable to it, because you know there will be a price to pay if you don't.

Got the flu? Thank the brew

Too much alcohol in any form weakens your immune system, making it easier than ever for you to get sick. It does this by:

1. *Interfering with the way your body absorbs and stores immune-boosting vitamins and minerals*
2. *Reducing the ability of your white blood cells to fight germs and infections*

You can't afford to get sick during finals week, so think before you overindulge!

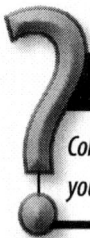

DID YOU KNOW?

Cold showers or hot coffee won't help sober you up. Time is the only factor. It takes your body one hour to eliminate the alcohol in one drink.

Energy drink + hard liquor ≠ an energetic drunk

Alcohol is a depressant. Caffeine is a stimulant. So that means that if you knock down an energy drink mixed with vodka, the caffeine will drown the effects of the alcohol, right? Wrong! Not only have studies shown that college students who consume energy drinks with alcohol drink more, but they also drink for longer periods of time, have higher blood-alcohol levels and are four times more likely to try to drive drunk. The stimulating effects of the energy drink can trick your brain into thinking you're sober when in fact you're drunk. In other words, you become an "awake" drunk.

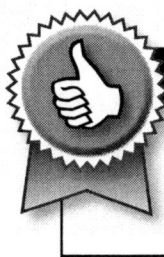

GOOD IDEA!

Always elect a designated driver. Being a responsible college student extends far beyond attending your classes. It means being responsible for your safety, too.

7 tips for safer, smarter drinking

1. ***Eat something before you drink***—*a meal with substance, not a garden salad! A big bowl of cereal with fruit or a grilled chicken sandwich with lots of veggies should do the trick. Food with substance helps "soak up" the alcohol and slow its absorption.*

2. ***Go light and slash the calories.***
   ✓ Wine spritzers are an easy way to reduce the alcohol content and overall calories. Mix 2 ounces of wine with 2 ounces of club soda.
   ✓ Dilute your drink with lots of ice
   ✓ Choose light versions when possible and take in 25% fewer calories.

3. ***Put a cap on it! Limit yourself to one or two drinks***

4. ***Know what a serving of alcohol really is:***
   ✓ 12 ounces of beer
   ✓ 5 ounces of wine
   ✓ 1.5 ounces of hard liquor

5. ***Drink slowly.*** *Your liver breaks down the alcohol from one drink in about an hour. If you give it too much to filter, it becomes overwhelmed and you become intoxicated.*

6. **Stay hydrated!** *For every alcoholic beverage, drink 8 ounces of water.*

7. **DO NOT get behind the wheel of a car after you've been drinking, and don't let your friends, either. Take their keys and take a cab.**

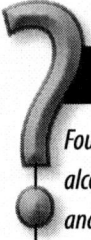

DID YOU KNOW?

Fourteen hundred college students from the ages of 18 to 24 die every year from alcohol-related unintentional injuries, including motor-vehicle crashes* Don't drink and drive! *Hingson et al., 2002

Uh-oh—I didn't listen. Now what?

Okay, so you had one too many drinks and now you're paying the price. Your first thought is to lie in bed all day, nurse your hangover and beg your roommate to pick you up a Chipotle burrito. That plan will leave you hanging on to your hangover even longer. Below you'll find a plan you can follow to help pick yourself up and get back on track. Your body (and your roommate) will thank you for it.

The 3-Step Day-After Forgiveness Plan

Step 1: Hydrate

Fill your water bottle and drink. Start with 16 ounces. Don't forget to check the color of your urine. If it's the color of the beer you drank last night, hydrate some more. If at some point you found yourself in the bathroom hugging the porcelain throne, be sure to replenish your electrolytes with coconut water or a sports drink like Gatorade.

Step 2: Remove butt from bed

The last thing you want to do is exercise, but it's the only thing that will make you feel better immediately. Take a brisk 20-minute walk or hop on the stair climber at the rec center. Do something, anything—just move! Don't forget to carry your water bottle with you and hydrate some more.

Step 3: *Nourish*

Be kind to your body today and feed it well. Here's a good plan:

- ✧ Breakfast: Eat a bowl of fortified cereal with skim milk (try to pass on the Lucky Charms and go for Whole Grain Total Raisin Bran instead).
- ✧ Lunch: Eat a nice big salad with lots of veggies, beans, a small portion of lean protein like baked chicken or fish and a whole-grain roll.
- ✧ Dinner: Try a big bowl of chicken-noodle or vegetable soup with half a sandwich.
- ✧ Snacks: Between meals, snack on fruit, nuts, string cheese or carrot sticks with hummus or peanut butter.

Good grades and a sexy body aren't likely when you overdo it on the alcohol. If you decide to drink, please be responsible.

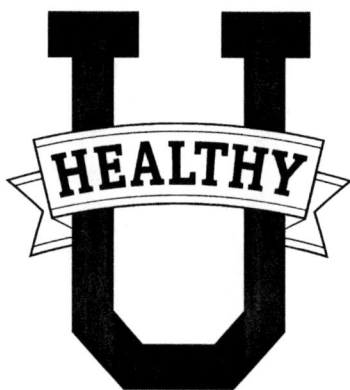

Secret 13

FEED YOUR BRAIN

What's in it for you?

✓ Learn what to eat to stay calm and focused

✓ Perk up your brain

✓ Learn what foods to eat for a better memory

✓ Stop falling asleep in class

Keep it light! Large meals equal heavy eyes

You really are what you eat. Whether it's leftover pizza or a bowl of grapes, what you eat has a direct effect on your body. Your memory, ability to concentrate and energy level depend largely on what you feed your face.

3 food factors for peak brain and body power

If you eat doughnuts for breakfast, skip lunch and fill your dinner plate with mounds of food, you'll probably find yourself slumped over in class, ready to fall asleep. The following three food factors will help pull you out of your slump and keep you awake. You've already learned some of this information from previous Secrets, but you'll find it helpful to have it all in one place.

? DID YOU KNOW?

Carbohydrates, when eaten in moderation, won't make you fat. Refined carbohydrates, like cookies and candy, have lots of calories and will cause weight gain if you eat too much of them, and you probably do. When was the last time you ate just one bite of a candy bar or had just one sip of soda?

Factor 1: What you eat

Carbohydrates

Carbohydrates are the preferred fuel source for your brain and can be thought of in two categories: brain-building and brain-draining. Brain-building carbs digest slowly, pumping a steady supply of glucose to your brain. Brain-draining carbs release a gush of sugar into your bloodstream, followed by a crash-and-burn effect. The end result is irritability, sleepiness and inability to focus. Use the table below to choose brain-building carbs.

Brain-Building Carbs:	Brain-Draining Carbs (simple sugars or sweets):
Whole-grain cereals, crackers, bread, pasta, oats, brown rice, etc. Fruit (fresh or frozen rather than juice) Legumes: dried beans, peas and lentils Milk and yogurt Vegetables	White bread, bagels Muffins, pastries, doughnuts White rice Sugary cereals Cookies Cakes Candy Frosting Kool-Aid and fruit drinks Soda Sweetened coffee drinks Sweet tea Sweeteners: table sugar, syrups, jams jellies, brown sugar, raw sugar

DID YOU KNOW?

Sugar doesn't give you energy or make you hyper. The opposite is true. Shortly after eating something with a lot of sugar, you'll start to feel sluggish and "foggy."

DID YOU KNOW?

If you're really craving something sweet like a piece of candy or cake, eat it after a meal to weaken the "serotonin effect."

In Secret 4, you learned that when you eat healthy, brain-building carbohydrates, the level of tryptophan in your body increases, producing enough serotonin to:

✓ Make you feel happy and calm

✓ Control your appetite

✓ Help you sleep better

✓ Improve your memory

✓ Help you focus, making learning easier

✓ Make you feel energetic

Some researchers believe that carbohydrate cravings signal a dip in your body's serotonin stores. This may explain why you sometimes crave cookies or other carbohydrate-rich foods in the late afternoon and evening or when you're feeling blue. This is your body's way of trying to boost its serotonin level so that it can feel better. You're craving brownies, but what you really need are starchy brain-building carbohydrates like whole-grain cereal, crackers and popcorn. Making the smart choice will give your body what it's craving (carbohydrates) without adding unnecessary sugars and calories.

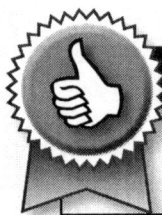

GOOD IDEA!

If you get hungry around bedtime, a bowl of oatmeal is a perfect brain-building carbohydrate to help you relax.

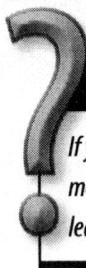

DID YOU KNOW?

If you go on a low-carb, high-protein diet, you'll probably crave carbohydrates even more. It's best to follow a healthy diet with a balance of brain-building carbohydrates, lean protein and healthy fat.

Protein:

The "fight or flight" chemicals that perk you up are dopamine, epinephrine and norepinephrine. They're made from the amino acid tyrosine, found in certain protein-rich foods. Eating a little protein with each of your meals helps you:

✓ Respond well to stress

✓ Stay alert

✓ Stay focused and energized

It's important to note that when you eat a meal with both protein and carbohydrate, like a chicken sandwich on whole-wheat bread, tyrosine will overpower tryptophan in the brain and you'll feel more alert and be ready to handle stress. If, on the other hand, you eat a non-protein (carbohydrate) meal, like a bowl of oatmeal, tryptophan will win and enter your brain. Now you're feeling happy and calm.

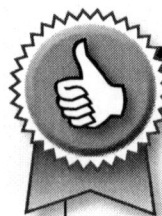

GOOD IDEA!

To stay alert during the day, be sure to eat some protein with your breakfast and lunch. How about a hard-boiled egg with breakfast and a veggie burger with your lunch?

Brain-building fats:

a. Polyunsaturated fats (omega 3 fatty acids):

Your brain is two-thirds fat, so it's important to eat enough fat. Your brain thrives on certain fats more than others, namely the omega 3 fatty acids DHA (docosahexaenoic acid) and EPA (eicosa-pentaenoic acid). ALA (alpha-linolenic acid) is another omega 3 fatty acid your body can convert into DHA, but not fully. ALA is healthy and worth including in your diet, but DHA and EPA are the best. DHA happens to be the main structural component in your brain, so it makes sense that a diet rich in DHA omega 3 fatty acids will produce a higher-functioning noggin. Fatigue, poor memory, mood swings and depression can result if you're not getting enough omega 3's in your diet. See the list below for foods rich in all three omega 3 fatty acids.

Foods rich in DHA and EPA omega 3 fatty acids	Foods rich in ALA omega 3 fatty acids
Herring	Chia seeds
Mackerel	Canola oil
Salmon	Flaxseed
Sardines	Flaxseed oil
Trout	Soybeans
Tuna	Soybean oil
	Omega 3 fatty acid-fortified eggs
	Pumpkin seeds
	Tofu
	Walnuts

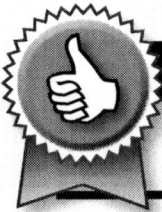

GOOD IDEA!

Eat some pumpkin seeds for a snack.

b. Monounsaturated fats:

Eat these fats to support healthy blood flow to your brain. They lower your total and LDL cholesterol (the "bad" cholesterol) levels. The best sources of monounsaturated fats are:

✓ Avocados

✓ Canola oil

✓ Nuts (also high in vitamin E, which preserves your memory)

✓ Olives/olive oil

✓ Peanut oil

✓ Seeds

✓ Sunflower oil

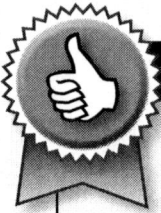

GOOD IDEA!

Swap the sour cream for a small scoop of guacamole on your nachos or burrito. Although it's considered a fruit, avocados are counted like a fat. Don't be afraid of them, because they're a healthy fat—two tablespoons of guacamole or two to three thin slices of avocado have 50 calories and 4.5 grams of fat (only 0.5-gram of saturated fat). Compare that with 50 calories and 5 grams of fat (3 grams of saturated fat) in two tablespoons of sour cream and 200 calories and 23 grams of fat (14.6 grams of saturated fat) in two tablespoons of butter.

Brain-draining fats: trans fats

Trans fats (trans fatty acids) are created when oil is turned into a solid fat during a process called partial hydrogenation. Trans fats are in many foods, such as commercial baked cakes, cookies and crackers. They're also in foods that are fried in partially hydrogenated oils such as chicken and french fries.

Trans fat make their way into your brain cells, line your brain-cell membranes and interfere with your thought processes. You would be wise to become an avid label reader and eliminate these fats from your diet completely. For more specific details on trans fats, refer back to *Secret 2: Get Smart, Eat Fat.*

B-vitamins and choline:

B-vitamins turn the energy from the foods you eat into energy you can use to get you through the day. Your brain isn't as sharp without B-vitamins. Choline belongs to the B-vitamin family and improves thought, memory and focus.

Name of B-vitamin	Food Sources	
Vitamin B1—Thiamin	Dairy products Enriched grains Fish Fruits Lean meats Legumes	Nuts and seeds Soybeans Vegetables Wheat germ Whole grains
Vitamin B2—Riboflavin	Cottage cheese Enriched grains Leafy greens Meat	Milk Whole grains Yogurt
Vitamin B3—Niacin	Eggs Enriched grains Fish Lean meats Legumes	Milk Nuts Poultry Whole grains
Vitamin B5—Pantothenic acid	Broccoli and other vegetables in the cabbage family Eggs Fish Lean beef	Legumes Milk and milk products Poultry Whole-grain cereals

Name of B-vitamin	Food Sources	
Vitamin B6—Pyridoxine	Fish and shellfish Fruits Leafy greens Legumes	Meats Poultry Whole grains
Vitamin B7—Biotin	Broccoli and other vegetables in the cabbage family Eggs Fish	Lean beef Legumes Milk and milk products Whole grain cereals
Vitamin B9—Folate/Folic Acid	Citrus fruits Leafy greens Legumes	Seeds Whole grains
Vitamin B12—Cobalamin	Animal products (meat, fish, poultry, shellfish, milk, cheese, eggs, yogurt) Fortified grains	
Choline	Egg yolk Liver Soybeans	Wheat germ Whole-wheat products

If you eat a balanced diet that's rich in fruits, vegetables, whole grains and legumes with moderate amounts of lean meats, fish and dairy products and small amounts of healthy fats like nuts, you'll have no problem getting your daily dose of B-vitamins. It's when you get into the habit of eating processed, refined foods and very little produce that you may lack these all-important vitamins.

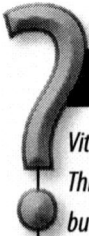

DID YOU KNOW?

Vitamin B-12 is found only in animal products and some fortified cereals (like Total). This vitamin helps form your red blood cells, maintain a healthy nervous system and build your DNA (your genetic material). If you're a vegan (a vegetarian who eats no animal products), you may want to consider eating a bowl of Total cereal every day or taking a multivitamin.

Antioxidants:

The more free radicals in your body that you can neutralize and get rid of, the better. Your body naturally eliminates some of them, but it can use some help. Eating foods high in antioxidants tips the scales in your favor. Antioxidants act like a broom in your body, sweeping up and eliminating free radicals.

The antioxidant level of food is measured using the ORAC scale (oxygen radical absorbance capacity). The higher the ORAC score, the more antioxidants a food has. Antioxidant-rich foods include those rich in:

✓ Vitamin A

✓ Vitamin C

✓ Vitamin E

✓ Polyphenols (found in colorful fruits and vegetables)

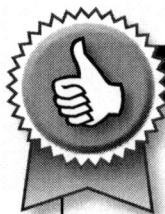

✓ Selenium

GOOD IDEA!

If you're looking for a hot beverage to sip on that doesn't have too much caffeine, try a cup of green tea. A 6-ounce serving of green tea has only 26 mg of caffeine—about the amount in a third of a cup of coffee—but lots of antioxidants!

Here are the top-scoring foods:

Top Scoring Antioxidant-Rich Foods

- Apples with skins
- Apricots (dried)
- Artichokes
- Asparagus
- Avocados
- Beans and legumes
- Beets
- Bell Peppers
- Berries
- Broccoli

- Cabbage
- Cherries
- Currants
- Figs
- Grapefruit
- Grapes
- Green leafy lettuce
- Guava
- Kiwi
- Mango

- Onions
- Oranges
- Peaches
- Pears
- Plums/Prunes
- Pomegranates
- Potatoes with skin *(sweet and white)*
- Radishes
- Raisins
- Spinach

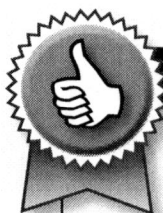

GOOD IDEA!

Good idea: Keep a stash of frozen blueberries in your freezer. They're cheaper and typically more nutritious than fresh blueberries.

Brain Berry Shake

(275 calories)

1 cup frozen blueberries

6 oz. low-fat plain or vanilla yogurt

6 oz. skim or soy milk

Place all ingredients in a blender and blend until smooth. Makes one serving.

Water:

Your brain is about 80% water. You learned how important proper hydration is to your body and brain in *Secret 9: Energize with H₂0*. But did you know that even mild dehydration can result in a decline in mental performance, raise your stress hormones and weaken your brain over time? Be sure to drink plenty of water throughout the day to keep your brain in top shape. For more information and fluid recommendations, refer back to Secret 9.

Factor 2: How often you eat

If it's extra energy and more focus you're after, it's critical to refuel every few hours. This includes the most important meal of the day: breakfast. To break the overnight fast that happens when you sleep, breakfast is a must. Breakfast doesn't have to be a big meal (in fact, it shouldn't be). A slice of whole-grain bread with peanut butter or a piece of fruit with a handful of almonds are great choices for breakfast. A random survey of students at Ohio State University revealed that 33% don't eat breakfast. Interestingly enough, the survey also showed that 32% of students acknowledged feeling sluggish throughout the day. You can't help but wonder if they are the same people who don't eat breakfast.

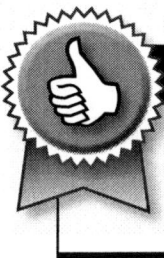

GOOD IDEA!

Don't skip meals. Always carry easy, portable foods with you just in case. An apple, a banana, a granola bar, dry cereal, string cheese, baby carrots, almonds and raisins are quick snacks you can easily toss into your bag.

If your blood-sugar level drops below a certain point, say after about four hours with no food, you can begin to experience symptoms of hypoglycemia (low blood sugar), such as:

- ✓ Hunger
- ✓ Shakiness
- ✓ Nervousness
- ✓ Sweating
- ✓ Dizziness or lightheadedness

- ✓ Sleepiness
- ✓ Confusion
- ✓ Difficulty in speaking
- ✓ Anxiety
- ✓ Weakness

To prevent low blood sugar and the low energy and brain function that follow, get into the habit of eating every few hours throughout the day, and never let more than four hours pass without eating something.

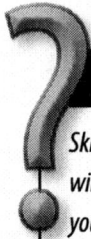

DID YOU KNOW?

Skipping meals will bring your metabolism to a screeching halt. This means your body will burn calories at a much slower rate, making it easier than ever to gain weight. If you're looking to stay slim and trim in college, you need to eat!

If there's one thing I learned about eating healthy in college, it's that I have to have a certain time schedule to eat or else, at midnight, I'm starving and looking for something to eat right before I go to bed.

—ANGELA, junior at John Carroll University

I lived in a house of college athletes. We were hungry all the time. Anything left in the fridge was fair game—even if it was pierogies or leftover spaghetti and meatballs at 7 a.m.

— VERONICA, recent graduate of Ohio State University

Factor 3: How much you eat

Large high-calorie meals take longer to digest and make you feel sleepy. Lighter meals with fewer calories keep you energized and give you peak mental focus.

You probably have to be at your sharpest during daylight hours, so breakfast, lunch and snacks should be light on calories but still satisfying. In other words, just because you're eating light doesn't mean you should go hungry.

In *Secret 17: Plan Your Plate*, you'll find Power Meal Plates™ to help you plan well-balanced meals and snacks. They do all the work for you and are:

✓ Calorie-controlled and satisfying

✓ Nutritious, with a balance of immune-boosting, brain-building and stress-busting foods

✓ Complete with the proper blend of carbohydrates, protein and fat to keep you sharp when you need to be and help you relax after a long day of classes

BRAIN-BUILDING POWER HABITS™!

✓ Eat only brain-building carbohydrates today. If you can't stop yourself from indulging in a brain-draining carb like soda or a cookie, be sure to eat or drink it after your meal to weaken the serotonin effect.

✓ Don't skip meals, especially breakfast. If you're in a hurry and have to eat on the go, grab a Kashi Honey Almond Flax bar and wash it down with 8 ounces of skim milk (226 calories, 54% carbohydrate, 26% protein, 20% fat).

✓ To rev up your brain in the morning, eat a light breakfast with some lean protein and brain-building carbohydrates (example: a three-egg-white omelet with 1 ounce of Cheddar cheese, a half-cup of black beans and a small banana).

✓ To get your B-vitamins, be sure to eat a few servings of whole grains today.

✓ Whether it's for breakfast or as a snack, find a way to eat an egg today to boost your choline (and your memory, too).

✓ Keep it light! Large meals equal heavy eyes.

✓ Sweep up the free radicals in your body with antioxidant-rich foods. Pick three from the list to include in your diet today.

✓ Write your own Brain-Building Power Habit™: _____

_____

_____

The Bottom Line

Small adjustments in what you eat and how you structure your meals can make you more alert and energized. Pick whichever Brain Building Power Habit(s)™ sound easiest and make your food work for you today! Don't forget to record it on your Power Habit™ Tracking Chart in the back of the book!

Secret 14

EAT TO AVOID THE FLU

What's in it for you?
✓ Miss fewer classes

✓ Feel more rested

✓ Have more energy!

Even the slightest deficiency of a single nutrient can make it tough to fight off infections

Your professor won't postpone the test because you got the flu, so why not do something to prevent yourself from getting sick in the fist place?

Your body is an amazing machine and comes equipped with a natural disease-fighting system, your immune system. It's armed with millions of "defenders"—specialized cells in your body called white blood cells. Certain foods boost your immune system, while others paralyze it. Even the slightest deficiency of a single nutrient can make it tough to fight off infections.

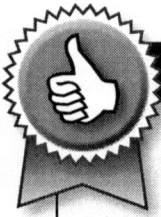

GOOD IDEA!

Flaxseed is a good source of brain-building, immune-boosting omega 3 fatty acids and fiber. The seeds can be eaten whole or ground, although your body absorbs the nutrients better in ground form. Add ground flaxseed to yogurt or oatmeal or sprinkle it on top of the jelly in your PB&J.

As a college student with a demanding schedule, you need to feed your body the right immune-boosting foods. Here are the most powerful ones you can get your hands on:

Vitamin A-Rich Foods *Antioxidant*	Apricots Asparagus Beet greens Broccoli Cantaloupe Carrots Cherries Corn	Green Peppers Kale Mangoes Nectarines Peaches Pink grapefruit Pumpkin Romaine Lettuce	Spinach Squash Sweet potatoes Tangerines Tomatoes Turnip/collard greens Watermelon
Vitamin C-Rich Foods *Antioxidant*	Berries Honeydew Papaya Broccoli Kale Peppers	Brussels sprouts Strawberries Cantaloupe Mangoes Snow peas Cauliflower	Nectarines Sweet potatoes Grapefruit Oranges Tomatoes
Vitamin B6-Pyridoxine	Fish and shellfish Fruits Leafy greens	Legumes Meats	Poultry Whole grains
Vitamin B9- Folate/ Folic Acid	Citrus fruits Leafy greens	Legumes Seeds	Whole grains
Vitamin E-Rich Foods *Antioxidant*	Broccoli Margarine Red peppers Carrots Mustard greens Spinach	Chard Nuts Sunflower seeds Fortified cereals Turnip greens	Mangoes Pumpkin Vegetable oils Papaya Wheat germ

Copper	Beans Fish	Nuts and seeds Organ meats (kidneys, liver)	Oysters and other shellfish Whole grains
Iron	Red meat Egg yolk Dark leafy greens (spinach, collards)	Poultry Beans, lentils, soybeans Liver	
Zinc	Beans Fortified cereals Oysters Beef (lean)	Milk Poultry Crab Nuts	Eggs Fish Tofu Wheat germ Yogurt
Omega 3 Fatty Acid-Rich Foods	**DHA/EPA-rich:** Herring Mackerel Salmon Sardines Trout Tuna	**ALA-rich:** Canola oil Flaxseed oil Soybean oil Chia Seeds Flaxseed Omega 3 eggs	Pumpkin seeds Soybeans Tofu Walnuts
Selenium-Rich Foods *Antioxidant*	Beans/legumes Beef Garlic Shrimp Brazil nuts Tuna	Brown rice Lobster Vegetables Chicken Whole grains	Cottage cheese Nuts/seeds Egg yolk Red snapper Poultry
Yogurt	Plain yogurt	Greek yogurt	Flavored yogurt
	Offers healthy bacteria to stimulate white blood cells		

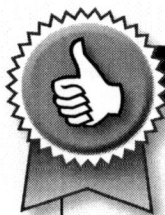

GOOD IDEA!

Eat a bowl of chicken soup if you feel like you're coming down with a cold.
There's a reason why Mom always made it for you when you were sick:
Chicken is a good source of vitamin B6, iron, zinc and selenium—
all immune boosters!

DID YOU KNOW?

Chia seeds are the same seeds used to grow the famous Chia Pets. They're edible and *very* nutritious. A good source of fiber and omega 3 fatty acids, chia seeds can be *eaten* just like flaxseeds, but they don't have to be ground in order to be absorbed. They even form a gel when mixed with liquid, acting as a thickener for drinks or smoothies.

8 ways to bust your immune system

1. *Eating too much sugar*

Sugar weakens your white blood cells and renders them defenseless against harmful germs and bacteria. Natural sugars, like those found in milk and fruit, are fine. It's the simple sugars you'll want to cut back on: soda, candy, pastries, cookies, fruit drinks, sweet teas, etc.

2. *Eating too much saturated fat and trans fats*

Both trigger inflammation in the body. Keep your saturated-fat intake low, and eliminate trans fats completely.

3. *Drinking too much alcohol*

Just like sugar, alcohol weakens your white blood cells' ability to destroy germs. Have a beer and your body also won't be able to use the nutrients from those immune-boosting foods above.

4. *Not getting enough sleep*

You may have noticed that when your sleep schedule is off thanks to deadlines, cramming during finals week or late-night parties, you're more likely to get sick. This is because lack of sleep causes inflammation in the body. To stay healthy, you should try to get from seven to nine hours of sleep every night.

5. *Not washing your hands often enough*

Your hands are simply crawling with germs. Washing your hands is the number one way to prevent these germs from entering your body and making you sick. Bottom line — wash them more than you do now.

6. *Lack of exercise*

   Regular exercise boosts the immune-system cells (called leukocytes) in your body, protecting you from illness.

7. *Carrying around excess body fat*

   Too many fat cells will trigger inflammation in the body, destroy healthy tissue and weaken your immune system.

8. *Too much stress*

   Short-term stress may help boost your immune system. When stress gets to be too overwhelming, however, your body pumps out a steady stream of stress hormones (called cortisol and adrenaline) that can suppress your immune system, making you extra-vulnerable to infection.

Immune-boosting meal and snack ideas

For more:	Try this:
Vitamin A:	Toss some beets onto your salad
Vitamin C:	Eat half a grapefruit with breakfast
Vitamin B6:	Choose romaine or spinach instead of iceberg lettuce for your salad
Folic acid:	Eat a bowl of bean soup or chili for dinner
Vitamin E:	Eat a handful of peanuts for a snack
Copper:	Ask for your sub on whole-grain bread
Zinc:	Eat a hard-boiled egg for a snack
Iron:	Snack on dry cereal like Frosted Mini-Wheats
Omega 3's:	Try baked salmon instead of baked chicken for dinner
Selenium:	Choose brown rice over white
Healthy bacteria:	Greek yogurt, 1 teaspoon of honey and a quarter-cup of blueberries

IMMUNE-BOOSTING POWER HABITS™!

✓ Eat at least 1½ cups of fruit and 2 cups of vegetables every day.

✓ Eat a 6-ounce container of yogurt as a snack.

✓ Sprinkle some crushed walnuts or 1 tablespoon of milled flaxseeds on your oatmeal.

✓ Choose salmon or tuna instead of beef or chicken.

✓ Schedule exercise into your day and make it a priority. Start by committing to three days a week and build from there.

✓ Get at least seven hours of sleep each night.

✓ Watch the added sugars in your diet, especially soda! Choose water instead.

✓ Write your own Immune-Boosting Power Habit™: _____

_____

_____

The Bottom Line

Your immune system will work for you if you treat and feed your body well. Choose as many Immune-Boosting Power Habits™ to practice as you'd like and start getting healthier right now. Don't forget to record it on your Power Habit™ Tracking Chart in the back of the book!

DON'T EAT YOUR STRESS, BEAT IT!

What's in it for you?

✓ Use your stress to get things done

✓ Stop eating your way through a stressful day

✓ Learn which foods beat your stress and which ones cause it

Don't dance around your stress, dance with it

Juggling exams, papers, deadlines and a part-time job can stress you out. A 2006 survey conducted by the University of Maryland revealed that the most commonly shared concerns among college students were:

✓ Making the kinds of grades you want (mentioned by 59%)

✓ Procrastination (47%)

✓ Studying effectively (45%)

✓ Managing time (44%)

✓ Pressure as a result of deadlines (40%)

✓ Preparing for exams (40%)

✓ Sleeping too little (39%)

✓ Remembering what you've read (39%)

✓ Stress from overload (35%)

Stress can be a good thing if you use it to your advantage. It pushes you to take action and get things done. As the deadline for that Psychology 101 paper quickly approaches and you find yourself feeling more and more stressed about finishing it, you need to face that stress head-on. Don't dance around your stress it—dance with it!

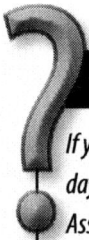

DID YOU KNOW?

If you feel stressed out, have difficulty sleeping, feel tired and sluggish during the day or have anxiety, you aren't alone. According to the American College Health Association's 2008 National College Health Assessment Survey, 87% of college students feel overwhelmed, 49% feel overwhelming anxiety, 90% don't get enough sleep and 45% feel tired, dragged out or sleepy during the day. A healthy diet can help you.

Dancing around your stress can take the form of any one of the following:

✓ Visiting your friends instead of studying for tomorrow's biology exam

✓ Writing that psychology paper with one hand and digging into a bag of chips with the other

✓ Watching yet another episode of *Jersey Shore* before reading your assigned history chapters

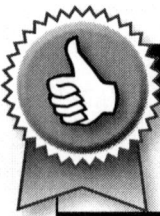

GOOD IDEA!

Make a list of all the ways you dance around your stress. You have to acknowledge the habit before you can break it.

Dancing with your stress means acknowledging that it's there, appreciating it and using it to your advantage to get things done. Sure, it's uncomfortable, which is why we try to avoid it, but that only makes it worse. Eating junk food to cope with your stress is a perfect example of trying to avoid it. And remember that eating some foods can make you feel even more stressed out.

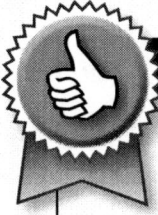

GOOD IDEA!

Spend five minutes in the morning to plan your day. When will you study? How much time will you spend working out? Will you have time to hang out with friends? How about sleep?

5 tips for dancing with your stress

The key is to have a plan in place to make stress work to your advantage. Any one of the following will work:

1. *Be proactive and eat satisfying, calorie-controlled, well-balanced meals and snacks throughout the day. Be sure to include plenty of foods rich in antioxidants, omega 3 fatty acids, B-vitamins and choline.*

2. *Spend five minutes in the morning planning your day.*

3. *When stress attacks, pick a positive way to cope with it. The wrong one is food. Here are some ideas that take no more than two minutes:*

   a. Move! Try 20 jumping jacks or 10 push-ups.

   b. Stretch! Sometimes just stretching your muscles can ease tension.

   c. Listen to calming music. Have it ready to go on your iPod for when you need it.

   d. Call a positive friend. Chances are he or she is feeling the same way. Don't call "Negative Nelly" or "Debbie Downer." You need to relieve your tension, not add to it.

e. Practice relaxation techniques:

    i. *Sit comfortably tall but relaxed in your chair and place your hand over your lower abdomen.*

    ii. *Inhale deeply, forcing your abdomen out. This fills the lower portion of your lungs with oxygen. Your chest should move only slightly. If you're sucking your stomach in and raising your chest, only the top parts of your lungs are working—this is shallow breathing. Oxygen flow isn't as great, which means your brain and muscles aren't being well-oxygenated and you'll hold on to more tension.*

    iii. *Exhale completely.*

    iv. *Repeat 10 times.*

Sometimes I dread going to my weekly yoga class (especially if I have an extra-crazy week), but once I get through it, I always feel less stressed and ready to focus on whatever project I have for that night.

    – ASHLEY, senior at North Carolina State University

4. **Get enough sleep.**

With all the demands of college life, sleep might seem like a luxury, not a necessity. But sleep deprivation aggravates stress! Be proactive and get enough sleep. It won't eliminate your stress, but it will help you cope with it. Aim for seven to nine hours each night. Get any more than nine hours and you may feel sluggish. Earplugs do wonders to drown out your snoring roommate.

5. ***If you find yourself turning to food to cope with your stress, have the right snacks on hand. The following will increase your tension:***

✓ Too much caffeine

✓ Sugary foods (candy, soda, cookies, snack cakes, etc.)

✓ Salty snack foods (chips, pretzels), which dehydrate your body and brain, leaving you fatigued

✓ High-fat meals (cheeseburgers, fries, mac-n-cheese, wings), which raise your stress-hormone levels and keep them high

✓ Alcohol

Give yourself permission to not be perfect.
... Doesn't that feel better?

Eat stress-busting foods often

Food:	How does it help your stress?	Sources of:		
B-vitamin-rich foods	✧ It maintains nerve and brain cells and converts the food you eat into energy you can use. ✧ You need it to make serotonin	Broccoli Fruits Poultry Cheese Leafy greens Seeds	Cottage cheese Lean meats Shellfish Eggs Legumes Soybeans	Enriched grains Milk Whole grains Fish Nuts Yogurt
Choline-rich foods	✧ Helps with memory ✧ Reduces inflammation	Egg yolk Liver	Soybeans Wheat germ	Whole-wheat products
Water	✧ Helps convert food into energy	Bottled water	Tap water	Flavored water (calorie-free)
Omega 3 fatty acid-rich foods	✧ Higher blood levels of omega 3 fatty acids have been linked to better mood	**DHA/EPA-rich:** Herring Mackerel Salmon Sardines Trout Tuna	**ALA-rich:** Canola oil Flaxseed oil Soybean oil Chia Seeds Flaxseed Omega 3 eggs Pumpkin seeds Soybeans Tofu Walnuts	
Whole grains	✧ Boosts serotonin— the "feel-good" brain chemical	Barley Brown rice Oatmeal	Popcorn Quinoa WG cereals	WG crackers WG bread WG pasta

Food:	How does it help your stress?	Sources of:		
Vitamin C-rich foods	✧ Contain antioxidants, which fight free radicals that get released when you're stressed	Berries Broccoli Brussels sprouts Cabbage Cantaloupe Cauliflower Grapefruit	Honeydew Kale Kiwi Mangoes Mustard greens Nectarines Oranges	Papaya Peppers Rutabagas Snow peas Strawberries Sweet potatoes Tomatoes
Vitamin E-rich foods	✧ Contain antioxidants, which fight free radicals that get released when you're stressed	Broccoli Carrots Chard Fortified cereals Mangoes Margarine	Mustard greens Nuts Papaya Pumpkin Red peppers Spinach	Turnip greens Sunflower seeds Vegetable oils Wheat germ
Magnesium	✧ Relaxes muscles and nerves ✧ Stress depletes this mineral	Beans Halibut Nuts	Seeds Soybeans	Spinach Wheat germ Whole grains
Selenium	✧ Repairs oxidative damage caused by stress	Beans/ legumes Beef Garlic Shrimp Brazil nuts Tuna	Brown rice Lobster Vegetables Chicken Whole grains	Cottage cheese Nuts/seeds Egg yolk Red snapper Poultry

5 stress-busting snacks

Snack 1:
¼ cup 1% cottage cheese (B-vitamins, selenium)

6 Triscuit crackers (whole grain, magnesium, choline, B-vitamins)

Snack 2:
1 small banana (B-vitamins)

½ ounce walnuts (B-vitamins, vitamin E, magnesium, omega 3 fatty acids)

Snack 3:
1 hard-boiled egg (choline, selenium, B-vitamins)

1 small orange (vitamin C, B-vitamins)

Snack 4:
1 tablespoon of peanut butter (B-vitamins, magnesium, vitamin E)

1 slice of whole-grain bread (whole grain, magnesium, choline, B-vitamins)

Snack 5:
1 Kashi cereal bar (whole grain, magnesium, choline, B-vitamins)

4 ounces of skim milk (B-vitamins)

STRESS-BUSTING POWER HABITS™!

✓ Make a list of all the ways you dance around your stress instead of dancing with it. Formulate a plan to tackle each one. What can you do instead?

✓ Instead of stuffing your face, do something positive (like calling a positive friend) to cope with your stress.

✓ Have healthy, stress-busting foods on hand in your dorm or apartment. Choose a nutritious and balanced snack if you must eat in response to stress.

✓ Get at least seven hours of sleep every night.

✓ Make time for exercise, especially if you expect to have an extra-stressful day.

✓ Realize that there are only 24 hours in the day. Don't put so much on your plate if you know there's no way you'll get it all done. Prioritize!

✓ Write your own Stress-Busting Power Habit™: _____

_____

_____

The Bottom Line

Stress is inevitable in college. Quit dancing around it and pick one or two Stress-Busting Power Habits™ to tackle it head-on. You'll save time and energy! If your stress is just too much to handle, seek help by visiting your campus counseling center. Don't forget to record your Power Habit™ on your Power Habit™ Tracking Chart in the back of the book!

Secret 16

EAT LEAN IN THE DINING HALL

What's in it for you?

✓ Save hundreds of calories

✓ Fit in more fiber in one easy step

✓ Boost your energy but not your jean size

You don't have to change your diet completely. Just tweak it.

I learned that an all-you-care-to-eat dining hall doesn't necessarily mean you should eat all you can. Best tip for not gaining weight in college: Watch your portions and be the slowest eater at the table.

—ALEXANDRA, sophomore at
Case Western Reserve University

Your dining hall is sort of like a restaurant. You can find healthy options like a salad bar and not-so-healthy ones like burgers and fries. Unfortunately, the unhealthy choices are often more enticing. How many times have you told yourself, "Today, I'm having a big salad," but forgot your vow the instant you caught a whiff of the fried chicken or set eyes on the chocolate-fudge brownie? It happens to everyone sometimes. The secret is to learn how to make a few changes that will keep you healthy without making you feel deprived.

You can save big on calories just by making some simple changes in your food choices. It takes only 500 extra calories a day to gain 1 pound in a week. The good news is it's not that difficult to spare yourself those extra calories. For example, you can save 500 calories simply by choosing the egg and cheese breakfast sandwich on an English muffin instead of the sausage, egg and cheese croissant and opting for brown rice over fried rice for dinner. Small substitutions will add up to big boosts in your energy level but not in your jean size.

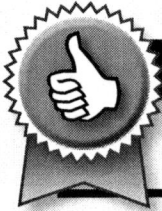

GOOD IDEA!

To control your portions, use a salad plate instead of a dinner plate.

This Secret gives you all the tools you need to find the silver lining in your dining hall. You can also use this information when you go to a restaurant or make meals at home. (The next Secret focuses on specific sample meals and specially designed Power Meal Plates™ so that you'll never be confused about what to eat again.)

Every dining hall has a silver lining.
You just have to look for it.

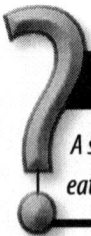

DID YOU KNOW?

A slice of cheese pizza can have up to 180 mg of calcium. Not bad! Just be sure to stop eating after one slice.

Give yourself an edge by getting familiar with food-preparation terms. The following descriptions let you know whether the food is healthy or fattening.

Beware of foods described like this:		Choose foods described like this:	
Au gratin	In cheese sauce	Baked	Grilled
Battered	Pan-fried	Braised	Poached
Béarnaise	Pastry	Broiled	Roasted
Breaded	Prime	Cooked in its own	Steamed
Buttered	Quiche	juices	Stir-fried
Cheesy	Rich		
Creamy	Sautéed		
Crispy	Scalloped		
Deep-fried	With gravy		
Double-crust	With mayonnaise		
Fried	With thick sauce		
Hollandaise	With white sauce		

My freshman year, I lived in a dorm that served all fried food after 8 p.m. My roommate and I would always go get snacks then. We both gained 25 pounds by Christmas! I'd always been heavier, so we decided we needed to make a change. We started eating healthier (baked chicken and veggies mostly) and working out. I ended up losing 75 pounds in a year and half! I haven't been this skinny since, like, elementary school!

—ELIZABETH, senior at Bowling Green State University

Lean your breakfast

Breakfast shouldn't always mean bacon and eggs or sausage and pancakes. The table below shows how easy it is to shave calories from your meals without compromising taste. You may be surprised to find that in many of the examples, you get more food by choosing the healthier option.

For BREAKFAST, instead of this:	Choose this:	And save this:
Home fries or hash browns	Red-skin potatoes, O'Brian potatoes	50 calories; 6 grams of fat; 1 gram of saturated fat
Medium blueberry muffin	Whole-wheat English muffin or half a whole-grain bagel with 1 tablespoon peanut butter	85 calories
Bacon, egg and cheese on a croissant	Egg and cheese on an English muffin	190 calories; 19 grams of fat; 8 grams of saturated fat; 0.5 grams of trans fat
Sausage, egg and cheese croissant	Egg and cheese on an English muffin	320 calories; 31 grams of fat; 12 grams of saturated fat; 0.5 grams of trans fat
Biscuits and gravy	Vegetable omelet or turkey egg white omelet	265 calories; 18 grams of fat; 3 grams of saturated fat; 8 grams of trans fat
Pork sausage	-Vegetarian sausage or -Turkey sausage	80 calories; 10.5 grams of fat; 4 grams of saturated fat; 0.1 grams of trans fat 75 calories; 9 grams of fat; 3.5 grams of saturated fat
White toast with butter	Whole-wheat toast with butter	Add 3 grams of fiber
2 Belgian waffles with fruit topping and whipped cream	Fruit and yogurt parfait with low-fat granola	670 calories; 62 grams of fat; 26 grams of saturated fat
French toast with ¼ cup maple syrup	Pancakes with fresh fruit and 2 tablespoons maple syrup	225 calories
Large plain bagel with cream cheese	Half a whole-grain bagel with peanut butter	125 calories
1 doughnut, cinnamon roll or Danish	Oatmeal with cinnamon and fresh berries	90 calories; 13.5 grams of fat; 2.5 grams of saturated fat
Sugary cereals with 2% or whole milk	Whole-grain cereals (like Kashi, Cheerios, Shredded Wheat) with skim or 1% milk	70 calories, 7 grams of fat; 12 grams sugar

Corned-beef hash	Scrambled eggs with grits or cream of wheat	90 calories, 9 grams of fat
1 strip of pork bacon	1 slice of Canadian bacon	3 grams of fat, 1 gram saturated fat
Large croissant	Half a whole-grain bagel or 2 slices whole-wheat toast	100 calories, 13 grams fat
Quiche	Omelet with beans, vegetables and 2 tablespoons cheese	160 calories, 11 grams of fat
Sausage, egg, cheese breakfast burrito	Egg, bean, salsa, cheese (just a sprinkle) breakfast burrito	160 calories; 18.5 grams of fat; 6 grams of saturated fat; 0.5 grams of trans fat
Venti Caffé Mocha with whipped cream	Tall non-fat Caffé Mocha with no whipped cream	240 calories, 15 grams of fat; 10 grams of saturated fat

DID YOU KNOW?

Just by choosing marinara sauce over cream sauce for your pasta, you'll save 120 calories and 13.5 grams of fat, and by choosing brown rice over fried rice, you'll save 200 calories and 12 grams of fat!

GOOD IDEA!

Blot your pizza with a napkin to remove the excess grease. To save on calories, instead of pouring dressing directly onto your salad, try putting it in a little cup and dipping your fork in before each bite.

Lighten your lunch and dinner

Lots of college students say they need to be even sharper and more focused in the afternoon and evening than in the morning. Probably because this is when a lot of students do the most studying. When you eat light and healthy, you'll have more energy to put into your work. Here's how to lighten your lunch and dinner with a few tweaks.

For LUNCH & DINNER, instead of this:	Choose this:	And save this:
-Creamy soups: cream of potato, cream of broccoli	Broth-based soups: vegetable soup, chicken-noodle soup	100 calories, 15 grams of fat
-Ramen noodle soup	-1 cup of chili or -1 cup of black bean soup	160 calories; 7.5 grams of fat 265 calories; 11.5 grams of fat
Alfredo or cream sauces on your pasta	Marinara sauce	120 calories, 13.5 grams of fat
Sausage and pepperoni cheese pizza	Vegetable cheese pizza	95 calories and 8 grams of fat per slice
Double cheeseburger on white bun	-Cheeseburger on whole-grain bun or -Veggie burger with lettuce and tomato on whole-grain bun	140 calories; 11 grams of fat; 5 grams of saturated fat; 1 gram of trans fat 190 calories; 14 grams of fat; 10 grams of saturated fat; 1.5 grams of trans fat
Breaded chicken sandwich on white bread	Grilled chicken sandwich on whole-grain bread	150 calories, 12 grams of fat
Loaded nachos	"Burrito Bowl" with chicken, rice, beans, salsa and lettuce	270 calories; 31 grams of fat; 4 grams of saturated fat; 0.5 grams of trans fat
Salad with iceberg lettuce, ranch dressing and croutons	Salad with romaine lettuce, balsamic vinaigrette and lots of vegetables	125 calories, 10 grams of fat
Fried rice	Brown rice	200 calories, 12 grams of fat
White rice	Brown rice	Add 4 grams of fiber
Beef hot dog	-Turkey hot dog or -Veggie hot dog (soy-based)	50 calories, 5 grams fat, 2.5 grams saturated fat 70 calories, 11 grams fat, 5 grams saturated fat

Chili cheese fries	Baked potato with chili, broccoli and a sprinkle of cheddar cheese	150 calories, 25 grams of fat
Regular pasta	Whole-grain pasta	Add 2 grams of fiber
Big bowl of macaroni and cheese	Half a bowl of macaroni and cheese, the other half cauliflower	265 calories; 10 grams of fat; 3 grams of saturated fat
White dinner roll	Whole-grain dinner roll	Add 2 grams of fiber
Fried/breaded fish	Grilled/baked fish	110 calories, 8 grams of fat
French fries	Baked, seasoned potato wedges, baked potato or sweet potato	350 calories, 23 grams of fat
Creamy salad dressings: ranch, blue cheese, thousand island	Oil-based salad dressings: balsamic vinaigrette, Italian, oil and vinegar	55 calories, 6 grams of fat
Mayonnaise on your sandwich	Hummus	65 calories, 8.5 grams of fat
Large chocolate chip cookie	Small oatmeal raisin or peanut butter cookie	100 calories, 4-6 grams of fat
Ice cream sundae	Fresh fruit salad	325 calories, 16 grams of fat
Big slice of cake with lots of frosting	-Small piece of cake with a thin layer of frosting or -Angel food cake with fresh fruit	150 calories, 5 grams of fat 150 calories, 17 grams of fat
Brownie	½ oz. of dark chocolate	100 calories, 5 grams of fat
16 oz. of soda, fruit punch, fruit drink or juice	Water with a twist of lemon or lime	200 calories

Slim down your snacks

Snacks are like mini-meals, so choose them wisely. Whenever possible, exchange high fat, sugar and salt bombs for real food.

For SNACK TIME, instead of this:	Choose this:	And save this:
Potato chips	Hummus with pita chips	40 calories, 9 grams of fat
Ice cream	Low-fat vanilla yogurt	50 calories, 6 grams of fat
Cookies	Granola bar	70 calories, 5 grams of fat
Pickles	Red pepper strips, cucumbers, baby carrots	650 mg of sodium
Saltine crackers	Triscuit Hint of Salt crackers	35 calories, 100 mg of sodium; add 2 grams of fiber
Candy: hard candy, caramels, etc.	-½ oz. dark chocolate or -Cluster of grapes	40 calories 60 calories
Butter Lover's popcorn (1 bag yields 10 cups)	Smart Balance Smart 'n Healthy popcorn (1 bag yields 15 cups)	40 calories, 16.5 grams of fat, 10 grams saturated fat, 745 mg sodium; add 7.5 grams of fiber!
Fruit snacks	Nuts and dried fruit	Add 2 grams of fiber
High-sugar granola bars (Sunbelt)	Less-sugar granola bars (Kashi)	2 grams of sugar; add 3 grams of fiber and 6 grams of protein

When I was a kid, my mom would always put Little Debbie Snack Cakes in my lunch. I grew up thinking that snacks meant Nutty Buddy Bars. It wasn't until I went away to college and started snacking on healthier things like apples and nuts that I realized what a difference it made in my energy level, especially in the afternoon when I needed a real pick-me-up.

—JASON, senior at Kansas State University

5 biggest dining-hall mistakes

1. ***Taking the all-you-can-eat buffet literally.***

   Solution: Take one plate, make one trip and be done with it.

2. ***Eating the same foods every day.***

   Solution: Go for variety and color. If you eat the same foods all the time, you're probably missing out on important vitamins and minerals.

3. ***Sitting too long.***

   Solution: When you're finished eating, get up and get out! The longer you sit there, the more tempted you'll be to go up for seconds.

4. ***Loading up on high-sugar sodas or juices or high-fat shakes.***

   Solution: Drink water. You can avoid gaining weight simply by cutting way back on calorie-rich beverages. Soda isn't the only culprit; juice has just as many calories!

5. ***Not speaking up.***

   Solution: Speak up! If you want your chicken plain, ask for it. If you'd rather have your turkey burger without the fried onions on top, ask for it.

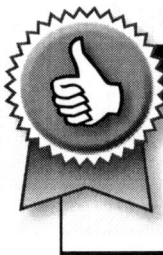

GOOD IDEA!

Try making a meal out of several side dishes. A baked potato, a serving of hot vegetables, a scoop of beans from the salad bar and a sprinkle of feta cheese and you have a delicious loaded potato.

LEAN DINING-HALL POWER HABITS™!

✓ Pass on the muffin for breakfast and fill up on a whole-grain English muffin or bagel with a smear of peanut butter instead.

✓ Fill your lunch or dinner plate with half veggies, a quarter lean meat, beans or soy and a quarter whole grain or starchy vegetable.

✓ Opt for whole-grain bread and pasta or brown rice instead of regular. To ease yourself into it, try asking for half whole-grain pasta or brown rice and the other half regular.

✓ Choose marinara or light garlic olive oil sauce instead of alfredo or other cream sauces.

✓ Choose broth-based soups over creamy soups for lunch and dinner.

✓ Slash 200 calories by drinking water with your meals instead of soda or fruit punch.

✓ Write your own Lean Dining-Hall Power Habit™: _____

_____

_____

The Bottom Line

Small tweaks in your food choices add up to big results! Get started by choosing one or two or three Lean Dining-Hall Power Habits™ from the list above, or get creative with your own Power Habit! Don't forget to record it on your Power Habit™ Tracking Chart in the back of the book!

Secret 17

PLAN YOUR PLATE

What's in it for you?

✓ Take the guesswork out of eating healthy

✓ Keep your calories in check

✓ Still enjoy your favorite comfort foods

All the work is done for you in this Secret. Everything you've learned up to this point comes together here. You have more than enough things to worry about in college; figuring out how to structure your meals doesn't have to be another one. Using the "Plan Your Plate" system will make it easy for you to stay on track with your healthy eating goals no matter how busy you are.

The key to eating healthy and avoiding weight gain in college is to have a plan. It doesn't have to be a big plan. Keep it simple and stick to it on most days and you'll be just fine.

The Power Meal Plates™

Here you'll find two specially designed Power Meal Plates™, one for breakfast and one for lunch or dinner. You'll also find many energizing good-for-you snack ideas, each with less than 250 calories.

When you follow the Power Meal Plates™ and snack ideas, you'll never go overboard on the portions, because each idea controls the amount of calories, fat, carbohydrate and protein you eat. The Power Meal Plates™ will also:

✓ Keep you calm and focused when you need to be at your sharpest

✓ Help control your stress during exam time

✓ Keep you from getting sick

✓ Stop weight gain before it has a chance to start

✓ Help you feel satisfied (no more grumbling stomach in class)

From now on, all you have to do is follow the Power Meal Plates™, plug in the foods available in your dining hall, dorm room or kitchen and enjoy! It's that's simple.

Daily rules of the "Plates":

If you want to get the most out of the Power Meal Plates™, strive to do the following every day:

✓ Eat three meals and two or three snacks

✓ Eat six servings of grains (make at least three of them whole grains)

✓ Eat five to seven ounces of meat/beans (and two servings of omega 3 fatty acid-rich fish each week)

✓ Drink 3 to 4 cups of milk or eat milk equivalents (four cups for 17- and-18 year-olds, 3 cups for ages 19 and over)

✓ Eat 2 cups of fruit

✓ Eat 2 to 3 cups of vegetables or more

✓ Include 6 teaspoons of healthy fats

✓ Eat omega 3 fatty acid-rich foods from one or two vegetarian sources

✓ Drink at least 48 ounces of water

✓ Limit your "Extras" to 300 calories or less per day

What about calories?

If you follow the guidelines in "Plan Your Plate," you shouldn't have to count calories (with the exception of keeping track of your Extras). To make this work best for you, determine how many calories you need every day to stay put at your current weight.

Your calorie level depends on your age, height, weight, activity level and gender and may be higher or lower than 2,000 calories a day. You can calculate it by using any of the online calorie calculators, like the one offered by the Mayo Clinic. You can find it at www.mayoclinic.com/ health/calorie-calculator/nu00598.

The Power Meal Plates™ and snacks provide about 1,900 to 2,100 calories a day assuming the above "rules" are followed. Add an extra snack or two or increase your portion sizes a bit if you need more calories or decrease them if you need less. Be careful not to eat fewer than 1,500 calories a day. If you're looking for a customized meal plan, visit www.mypyramid.gov.

This book is a guide to get you started and to keep you on the right track. It makes you aware of what you're putting in your mouth. College students gain weight because they eat too much, don't exercise enough or both. Calories sneak into your diet, portion sizes get bigger, you find yourself eating "just because," time isn't being set aside for a little exercise, and before you know it, the only clothes that fit are your sweat pants. Unfortunately, it's easy to gain weight and challenging to get rid of it. Not to worry. Awareness and healthy food will help you to detour college weight gain.

If you're looking for a customized meal plan or if you have unique dietary restrictions, your campus health center can help. Most universities employ a registered dietitian (RD) at the health center who's specially trained in food and nutrition.

The food lists

To make it even easier, a chart of foods with portion sizes is provided below for you to plug into the Power Meal Plates™. With the exception of the Extras, you're already familiar with these lists because they were covered by previous Secrets.

Don't want to weigh or measure your food? You don't have to! The portion sizes are compared to common objects like a baseball, a golf ball and a tennis ball so you won't have to worry about measuring. Just eyeball it. The goal of Secret 17 is to make this so simple that you can eat healthy, energizing meals from here on out.

Let's say you woke up too late to catch breakfast in the dining hall or you couldn't make it to dinner because you had to get that paper finished. Toward the end of this Secret, you'll find quick, healthy and balanced menus for breakfast, lunch and dinner that you can throw together in a snap so you won't have to rely on the nearest, fastest food. You'll also find sample meals and a full-day sample menu.

At the end of the day, it boils down to choices. Ultimately, it's you who has to make the better choice. Will you sometimes choose the french fries over the steamed vegetables? Sure. But as long as you opt for the healthier fare the majority of the time, you'll succeed in maintaining your current weight and may even drop a few pounds without even trying. You'll be pleasantly surprised when your taste buds change and you actually prefer the chicken Caesar salad to the hot wings!

> Who needs the "freshman 15" when you can gain the "freshmen 20"? Me!!! Now, as a senior, my freshman year is long gone and so are the pounds. With a balanced unrestricted diet and appropriate exercise, all I kept from that year were the memories.
>
> —JESSICA, senior at Penn State University

A note on beans

Beans count as a Meat & Bean and also as a Starchy Vegetable; you only need to count them once, though. For example, if you add black beans to your lunch salad, don't count it as both a Meat & Bean and a Starchy Vegetable. If you're a vegetarian or rarely eat meat, you may want to count it as a Meat & Bean. If, on the other hand, you had a piece of grilled chicken on that salad, you'd count the beans as a Starchy Vegetable.

A note on nuts, seeds and nut butters:

Nuts, seeds and nut butters count as both a Meat & Bean and a Healthy Fat. If you eat a peanut butter sandwich for lunch (with 2 table-spoons of peanut butter), this counts as 2 ounces of Meat & Beans and four teaspoons of Healthy Fat.

A note on the Extras:

The Extras include everything else, such as: condiments, sweets, soda, alcohol, potato chips, etc. This is the group that will get you into trouble if you're not careful, so keep track of them. You can also use your Extras if you want to eat more of a certain food group. Let's say you've already eaten six servings of grains today but you really have a taste for a Kashi Oatmeal Dark Chocolate cookie, which counts as two servings of grains. Should you deny yourself the cookie? No way! Go for it, but subtract it from your Extras.

Based on a 2,000-calorie-a-day meal plan, only 250 to 300 calories should come from Extras.

A note on naturally fatty foods

Pay attention to the total fat content of each meal, including healthy fat. For example, if you're using a full-fat dressing on your salad, think twice before adding cheese. If you really want the cheese, go for it, but use a lower-fat salad dressing. On the other hand, if you had a virtually fat-free breakfast of egg whites, toast and fruit, it's perfectly okay to have a little extra fat at lunch. It's all about balance.

Foods naturally containing fat include:

✓ Beef
✓ Pork
✓ Fatty cuts of meat (t-bone, tenderloin, porterhouse, brisket, rib-eye, flank, ribs, blade)
✓ Eggs

✓ Nuts and seeds

✓ Nut butters

✓ Cheese and other fuller-fat dairy products like cream, ice cream and 2% or whole milk

✓ Any Extra food that contains fat (e.g., chocolate, creamy salad dressings, mayonnaise, sour cream)

A note for vegetarians

No need to worry if you're a vegetarian. You'll notice that each of the food groups below has options for vegetarians and even vegans. The symbol 🍎 means the food is suitable for most vegetarians, and the symbol ▼means the food is vegan-friendly. *Secret 20: Vegetarian 101* describes the five types of vegetarians and offers important need-to-know information for those interested in adopting a vegetarian lifestyle and for those already living one.

A note on balance

Some days you'll eat more meat, and on other days you may have an extra serving or two of bread. On the weekends you might go overboard on pizza. It's okay! What matters is how well you practice balance over a seven-day period. So you ate three slices of pizza on Saturday—just behave yourself over the next few days and it'll all even out. Eating healthy isn't an all-or-nothing game. It's not about being a perfect eater; it's about being a better eater. In the end, it all comes down to balance.

* Foods naturally containing fat ♥ Omega 3 fatty acid-rich foods 🍎Vegetarian ▼Vegan

Meat & Beans			
Food	**One portion equals:**	**Counts as:**	**It's the size of:**
Beans: 🍎▼ Black, pinto, navy, soy♥, lentils, etc.	¼ cup	1 oz.	Egg
Eggs* 🍎 (omega 3 fatty acid-enriched♥)	1 whole egg 2 egg whites	1 oz.	
Fish/seafood (♥ depending on variety)	3 oz.	3 oz.	Checkbook

Meat & Beans

Food	One portion equals:	Counts as:	It's the size of:
Hummus 🍎▼	2 tablespoons	1 oz.	Golf ball
Meat*: beef, pork	3 oz.	3 oz.	Deck of cards/iPhone
Nuts and seeds* 🍎▼ Peanuts, walnuts▼, pecans, almonds, flaxseed▼, chia seeds▼, sunflower seeds, etc.	½ oz.	1 oz.	-2 tablespoons flaxseed, chia seeds or sunflower seeds -Small handful nuts
Nut butters* 🍎▼	1 tablespoon	1 oz.	Chocolate truffle
Protein powder Soy, rice, pea, hemp 🍎▼ Whey 🍎	1 standard scoop (from container)	3 oz.	
Poultry	3 oz.	3 oz.	Deck of cards/iPhone
Soups:	1 cup lentil soup 🍎▼ (vegetable broth; no meat)	2 oz.	
	1 cup bean soup/chili 🍎▼ (vegetable broth; no meat)	2 oz.	
	1 cup bean soup/chili (with meat)	2 oz.	
Soy	¼ cup tofu▼ 🍎▼	2 oz.	
	¼ cup soybeans▼ 🍎▼	1 oz.	
	2 breakfast links 🍎	1 oz.	
	1 breakfast patty 🍎	1 oz.	
	1 veggie burger 🍎	2 oz.	
	2/3 cup soy crumbles (Boca or MorningStar) 🍎	2 oz.	
	¼ cup dry TVP (textured vegetable protein) 🍎▼	2 oz.	
	4 MorningStar Meal Starter Strips 🍎▼	1 oz.	
	Note: To see if breakfast links, patties and veggie burgers are vegan-friendly, check nutrition label. Many contain eggs and milk.		

DID YOU KNOW?

Eating more protein won't build more muscle or make you stronger.

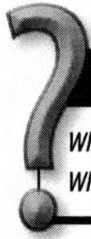

? DID YOU KNOW?

When milk is coagulated to make cheese, whey is the liquid product that's formed. Whey is a high-quality protein commonly found in protein powders.

Grains

All are vegetarian 🍎   Check label to see if vegan-friendly ▼

Food	One portion equals:	Counts as:	It's the size of:
Bread	1 slice	1 oz.	CD
Cereal (cold)	1 cup flakes or rounds ¼ cup granola ¼ cup Grape-Nuts	1 oz.	Baseball Egg Egg
Cereal (hot)	½ cup cooked oatmeal, grits, cream of wheat	1 oz.	Tennis ball
Crackers	WG: 5 whole-wheat crackers WG: 2 rye crispbreads 7 Saltines	1 oz.	
English Muffin	Half a muffin	1 oz.	
Granola bar	1 bar (1.2-oz size)	1-2 oz.	
Pancake/waffle	1 each	1 oz.	CD
Pasta, rice, barley, quinoa, couscous, other hot cooked grains	½ cup cooked	1 oz.	Tennis ball
Pita	1 mini-pita, 4" diameter (6" pita = 2 oz.)	1 oz.	
Popcorn (94% or more fat-free)	3 cups (1 bag microwave popcorn = 4 oz.)	1 oz.	
Roll	1 each	1 oz.	Yo-yo
Tortilla	1 small (6" diameter)	1 oz.	
Wheat germ	¼ cup	1 oz.	Egg
Whole-grain cookie (Kashi)	1 cookie	2 oz.	
Whole-grain tortilla chips	½ oz.	1 oz.	Handful

Milk

Food	One portion equals:	Counts as:	It's the size of:
*Cheese ᕯ (regular or soy▼)	1½ oz. hard cheese: Cheddar, mozzarella, Swiss, Parmesan 1 slice hard cheese 1/3 cup shredded 1 cup cottage cheese	1 cup ½ cup 1 cup ½ cup	6 stacked dice
Milk (1% or skim) (cow ᕯ; rice, almond or soy▼)	8 oz.	1 cup	
Yogurt (low-fat) (regular ᕯ or soy▼)	8 oz.	1 cup	

Fruit
All are vegetarian ᕯ   All are vegan ▼

Food	One portion equals:	Counts as:	It's the size of:
Fresh fruit	1 cup	1 cup	Baseball
Dried fruit	½ cup	1 cup	Tennis ball
100% fruit juice	8 oz.	1 cup	

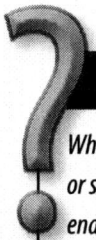

DID YOU KNOW?

Wheat germ is actually one of the layers of the whole grain kernel. It's the embryo, or sprouting section of the seed. The whole grain kernel is made up of the bran, endosperm and germ. The germ contains fiber, protein, iron, vitamin E, zinc, magnesium, phosphorus and some B-vitamins. It can be sprinkled on your cottage cheese, yogurt or hot cereal or added to your smoothie

Non-Starchy Vegetables
All are vegetarian 🍎   All are vegan ▼

Food	One portion equals:	Counts as:	It's the size of:
Fresh or frozen vegetables	1 cup	1 cup	Baseball
Raw leafy greens: spinach, romaine, watercress, dark green leafy lettuce, endive, escarole	2 cups	1 cup	2 baseballs
Vegetable soup (with ½ cup vegetables)	1 cup	½ cup	
Vegetable juice	8 oz.	1 cup	

Starchy Vegetables
All are vegetarian 🍎   All are vegan ▼

Food	One portion equals:	Counts as:	It's the size of:
Beans: Black, pinto, navy, soy♥, lentils, etc.	1 cup	1 cup	Baseball
Corn	1 cup	1 cup	Baseball
Peas	1 cup	1 cup	Baseball
Potatoes	1 cup 1 medium	1 cup	Baseball Computer mouse

Healthy Fats
All are vegetarian 🍎   All are vegan (Check salad dressing label) ▼

Food	One portion equals:	Counts as:	It's the size of:
Avocados Guacamole	Half a medium ½ cup	3 teaspoons 3 teaspoons	Tennis ball
*Nuts and seeds: peanuts, walnuts♥, pecans, almonds, flaxseed♥, chia seeds♥, sunflower seeds, etc.	½ oz.	1½ teaspoons	-2 tablespoons flaxseed, chia seeds or sunflower seeds -Small handful nuts
Nut butters	1 tablespoon	2 teaspoons	Chocolate truffle

Healthy Fats

All are vegetarian ♣   All are vegan (Check salad dressing label) ▼

Food	One portion equals:	Counts as:	It's the size of:
Vegetable oils: canola♥, corn, flaxseed♥, olive, peanut, soybean♥, sunflower	1 teaspoon	1 teaspoon	Postage stamp
Olives	8 large	1 teaspoon	
Salad dressings (non-creamy)	2 tablespoons	2 teaspoons	

Extras

Food	Portion size:	Calories:
Alcohol: Beer Wine Liquor	12 oz. 5 oz. 1 ½ oz.	145 105 100
*Bacon	1 medium slice	50
*Butter/margarine	1 pat/ 1 teaspoon	35
*Chocolate: Hershey's Kisses	2 Kisses	50
*Cookies	1 medium (e.g., Chips Ahoy, Oreo)	50-100
Condiments: Barbecue sauce *Creamy salad dressings Ketchup Salsa *Mayonnaise *Sour cream	1 tablespoon 1 tablespoon 1 tablespoon ¼ cup 1 tablespoon 1 tablespoon	25 75 20 20 50 25
*Cream (coffee cream)	1 tablespoon	20
*French fries	2.5 oz. (small order at McDonalds's)	230
Graham Crackers	1 sheet	60
*Gravy	¼ cup	30
*Ice cream	½ cup	130
*Potato chips	1 oz.	150

Extras		
Food	**Portion size:**	**Calories:**
Pretzels	1 oz.	110
Sauces: Marinara *Alfredo	 ½ cup ½ cup	 80 200
*Sausage	1 link	80
Soda	12 oz.	150
Sweeteners: Agave nectar Honey Jam/jelly Sugar (white, brown, raw) Syrup (pancake, other)	 1 tablespoon 1 tablespoon 1 teaspoon 1 teaspoon 1 tablespoon	 60 60 20 15 50

Breakfast Power Meal Plate™ and Sample Menus:
Breakfast

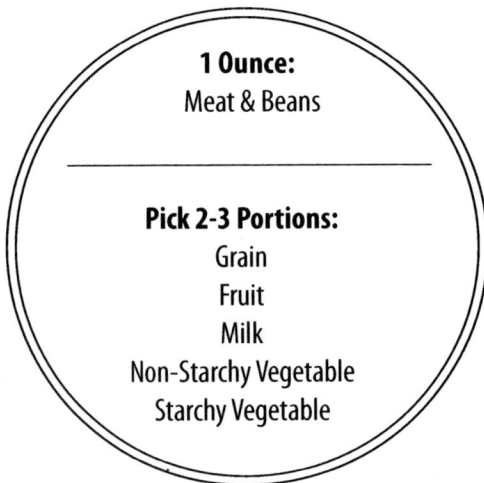

1 Ounce:
Meat & Beans

Pick 2-3 Portions:
Grain
Fruit
Milk
Non-Starchy Vegetable
Starchy Vegetable

+ 1 Portion of Healthy Fat
(Optional)

Minimum Daily Targets:

✓ 2-3 cups vegetables

✓ 2 cups fruit

✓ 6 ounces grains (at least three of them whole grains)

✓ 3-4 cups milk/milk products

✓ 5-7 ounces meat or beans (two servings omega 3-rich fish/week)

✓ 6 teaspoons of healthy fats

✓ 1-2 vegetarian sources of omega 3 fatty acid-rich foods

✓ 48 ounces of water

Sample Breakfasts	Category	Calories
1 cup cooked oats 1 cup strawberries 1 hard-boiled egg 1 tsp brown sugar	2 Grains 1 Fruit 1 oz. Meat & Beans Extra (15 calories)	300
1 soy sausage patty 8 oz. low-fat vanilla yogurt ¼ cup low-fat granola 1 cup blueberries	1 oz. Meat & Beans 1 Milk 1 Grain 1 Fruit	435
1 oz. Cheerios 8 oz. skim milk 1 small banana 1 tbsp peanut butter 1 tbsp cream for coffee	1 Grain 1 Milk 1 Fruit 1 oz. Meat & Beans; 2 tsp Healthy Fat Extra (20 calories)	395
2 egg whites ½ cup black beans 1 slice whole-wheat toast 1 pat butter 8 oz. skim milk	1 oz. Meat & Beans ½ Starchy Vegetable 1 Grain Extra (35 calories) 1 Milk	380
"Think Tank Shake" 8 oz. skim milk 1 cup berries 14 baby carrots 1 tbsp peanut butter	1 Milk 1 Fruit 1 Vegetable 1 oz. Meat & Beans; 2 tsp Healthy Fat	275
2 pancakes 2 tbsp maple syrup 8 oz. skim milk 1 egg	2 Grains Extra (100 calories) 1 Milk 1 oz. Meat & Beans	375

Lunch/Dinner Power Meal Plate™ and Sample Menus:

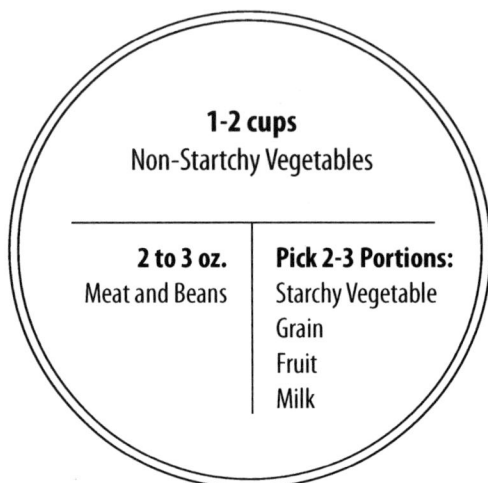

1-2 cups
Non-Startchy Vegetables

| **2 to 3 oz.** Meat and Beans | **Pick 2-3 Portions:** Starchy Vegetable Grain Fruit Milk |

+ 1 Portion of Healthy Fat
(Optional)

Minimum Daily Targets:

- ✓ 2-3 cups vegetables
- ✓ 2 cups fruit
- ✓ 6 ounces grains (at least three of them whole grains)
- ✓ 3-4 cups milk/milk products
- ✓ 5-7 ounces meat or beans (two servings omega 3-rich fish/week)
- ✓ 6 teaspoons of healthy fats
- ✓ 1-2 vegetarian sources of omega 3 fatty acid-rich foods
- ✓ 48 ounces of water

DID YOU KNOW?

An average-size slice of original-crust cheese pizza counts as 1 cup of milk and 2 ounces of grains.

DID YOU KNOW?

One cup of macaroni and cheese (made from a packaged mix) counts as 2 ounces of grains and a half-cup of milk.

Instead of this lunch/dinner	A better lunch/dinner	The BEST lunch/dinner	Category	Calories	Calories saved with the BEST choice
SALAD BAR! Chef's salad with creamy salad dressing (e.g., ranch)	Chef's salad with oil-based salad dressing and half the cheese	2 cups Romaine lettuce or spinach 1 cup tomatoes, cucumbers, red peppers 3 oz. tuna ½ cup chickpeas 1 cup fresh pineapple 1 whole-grain dinner roll 2 tbsp balsamic vinaigrette	1 Vegetable 1 Vegetable 3 oz. Meat & Beans 1/2 Starchy Vegetable 1 Fruit 1 Grain 2 tsp Healthy Fat	570	290
PIZZA! 2 slices of pepperoni pizza	1 slice of pepperoni pizza	1 small slice veggie cheese pizza 1 side salad 1 cup chopped broccoli 3 oz. grilled chicken strips 2 tbsp Italian dressing 1 small apple	1 Milk 1 Grain 1 Vegetable 1 Vegetable 3 oz. Meat & Beans 2 tsp Healthy Fat 1 Fruit	460	65
PASTA! Pasta with cream sauce	Small side of whole-grain pasta with cream sauce and baked chicken	1 cup whole-grain pasta ½ cup marinara sauce 3 oz. grilled salmon 1 cup cauliflower Kashi oatmeal cookie	2 Grains Extra (80) 3 oz. Meat & Beans 1 Vegetable Extra (130)	560	160
BURGERS! Cheeseburger with french fries	Cheeseburger or turkey burger with baked potato or side of veggies	1 veggie burger 1 slice of cheese 1 whole-wheat bun 1 tbsp ketchup 8 oz. Low Sodium V8 Juice Medium baked potato ¼ cup salsa	2 oz. Meat & Beans ½ Milk 2 Grains Extra (20 calories) 1 Vegetable 1 Starchy Vegetable Extra (20 calories)	600	80

Instead of this lunch/dinner	A better lunch/dinner	The BEST lunch/dinner	Category	Calories	Calories saved with the BEST choice
SUBS! A footlong cold-cut sandwich on white bread with regular potato chips	6" cold-cut sandwich on whole-grain bread with SunChips	6" chicken breast sub: 3 oz. grilled chicken Whole-grain bread Lettuce, tomato 4 large sliced olives Oil and vinegar 14 baby carrots	3 oz. Meat & Beans 3 Grains Garnish ½ tsp Healthy Fat 1 tsp Healthy Fat 1 Vegetable	500	220
MEXICAN! Chipotle-style burrito	Half a Chipotle-style burrito	Chipotle-style burrito bowl: 3 oz. steak or chicken ½ cup brown rice ½ cup black beans ¼ cup salsa 2 cups lettuce 1 cup fajita-style vegetables ½ cup guacamole	3 oz. Meat & Beans 1 Grain ½ Starchy Vegetable Extra (20 calories) 1 Vegetable 1 Vegetable 3 tsp Healthy Fat	535	190
ASIAN CUISINE! General Tso's chicken over fried rice	Half-portion of General Tso's chicken over brown rice	1 cup brown rice with ½ cup mandarin oranges 2 cups steamed broccoli 3 oz. pan-fried tofu 1 tsp oil 1 tsp light-sodium soy sauce 2 Hershey's Dark Chocolate Kisses	2 Grains ½ Fruit 2 Vegetables 3 oz. Meat & Beans 1 tsp Healthy Fat Extra (no calories) Extra (50 calories)	570	140
BALLPARK FOOD! A chili dog with cheese and an ice cream sundae for dessert	A chili dog without cheese and ½ cup ice cream for dessert	Veggie dog or turkey dog 1 whole-grain hot dog bun ½ cup chili 1 cup grapes 1 cup red pepper strips ½ cup ice cream	1 oz. Meat & Beans 1 Grain 1 oz. Meat & Beans 1 Fruit 1 Vegetable Extra (130 calories)	550	575

Yummy Comfort-Food Substitutions

Instead of this traditional comfort food	Try this healthier comfort food	Category	Calories	Calories saved
MACARONI & CHEESE!	1 cup whole-grain macaroni 1½ oz. of Cheddar cheese 1 cup cauliflower ½ cup edamame (soybeans)	2 Grains 1 Milk 1 Vegetable 2 oz. Meat & Beans	500	155
MEATLOAF, MASHED POTATOES & GRAVY	½ cup mashed potatoes 3 oz. turkey meatloaf 1 cup green beans ½ oz. slivered almonds 1 whole-grain dinner roll 1 cup cantaloupe 1 pat butter	½ Starchy Vegetable 3 oz. Meat & Beans 1 Vegetable 1 oz. Meat & Beans; 1 ½ tsp Healthy Fat 1 Grain 1 Fruit Extra (35 calories)	485	170
TOMATO SOUP & GRILLED CHEESE	**GOOD PRE-TEST MEAL 1 cup vegetable soup (with ½ cup vegetables) Half a whole-wheat pita 3 oz. tuna 1 tbsp olive-oil mayo ½ cup kidney beans	½ Vegetable 1 Grain 3 oz. Meat & Beans Extra (50 calories) ½ Starchy Vegetable	440	260
CHILI CHEESE FRIES!	1 medium baked potato 1 cup chili 1 tbsp sour cream 1 cup steamed broccoli	1 Starchy Vegetable 2 oz. Meat & Beans Extra (25 calories) 1 Vegetable	445	165
FRIED FISH & CHIPS	**GOOD PRE-TEST MEAL 3 oz. grilled salmon 1 medium sweet potato 1 tsp brown sugar 1 cup asparagus spears (about 10) Balsamic vinegar and 1 tsp olive oil ½ cup whole-grain rice pilaf	3 oz. Meat & Beans 1 Starchy Vegetable Extra (15 calories) 1 Vegetable 1 tsp Healthy Fat 1 Grain	490	590

Last year I drank a hot chocolate every day. Comfort food, yes. Good for my figure, no!

—ROSE, sophomore at the University of Louisville

Energizing Snacks

Put a healthy snack together in a snap by pairing choices from any two to three of the following categories. Pay attention to the serving sizes for snacks because they're smaller for a couple of the categories.

Category	Snack serving size
Meat & Beans	1 oz.
Grains	1 portion
Milk	Half- portion
Fruit	1 portion
Vegetables (non-starchy and starchy)	1 portion
Healthy Fat	1 portion

Energizing Snack	Category	Calories
5 Triscuit crackers ½ cup low-fat cottage cheese	1 Grain ¼ Milk	180
1 small banana 1 tbsp peanut butter	1 Fruit 1 oz. Meat & Beans; 2 tsp Healthy Fat	175
1 hard-boiled egg 1 cup orange sections	1 oz. Meat & Beans 1 Fruit	160
4 oz. low-fat vanilla yogurt ½ cup blueberries 2 tbsp Grape-Nuts cereal	½ Milk ½ Fruit ½ Grain	190
1 Honey Almond Flax Kashi bar 4 oz. skim milk	1 Grain ½ Milk	183
1 oz. whole-grain cereal 4 oz. skim milk	1 Grain ½ Milk	145
1 small apple ¾ oz. Cheddar cheese (size of 3 dice)	1 Fruit ½ Milk	160
1 Quaker Chocolate Crunch rice cake 1 tbsp almond butter	1 Grain 1 oz. Meat & Beans; 2 tsp Healthy Fat	160

Energizing Snack	Category	Calories
2 tbsp raisins 1 tbsp dark-chocolate chips ½ oz. peanuts	¼ Fruit Extra (70 calories) 1 oz. Meat & Beans; 1½ tsp Healthy Fat	200
¼ cup refried beans 1 small tortilla (6" diameter)	1 oz. Meat & Beans 1 Grain	150
8 oz. Low Sodium V8 Juice 1 string cheese	1 Vegetable ¾ Milk	130
½ cup baby carrots 2 tbsp hummus 5 Triscuit crackers	½ Vegetable 1 oz. Meat & Beans 1 Grain	175
¼ cup guacamole ½ oz. whole-grain tortilla chips	1½ tsp Healthy Fat 1 Grain	230
1 Kashi Oatmeal Cookie 4 oz. skim milk	2 Grains ½ Milk	175
English Muffin Pizza: -1 Hearty Grains Whole Wheat English Muffin (toasted) -¼ cup pizza sauce -2 tbsp shredded part-skim mozzarella cheese *Top English muffin with sauce and cheese and microwave until cheese melts (about 1 minute)*	2 Grains Extra (45 calories) 1/3 Milk	215
1 cup cherry tomatoes and red bell pepper slices ¼ cup edamame 1 whole-grain mini bagel	1 Vegetable 1 oz. Meat & Beans 1 Grain	215

Quick and Healthy Dorm-Room Meals

3-minute "no time for breakfast" ideas

Fast breakfast idea	Category	Calories
1 slice Cheddar cheese (1 oz.) 1 small apple ½ oz. walnuts 1 oz. Cheerios	½ Milk 1 Fruit 1 oz. Meat & Beans; 1½ tsp Healthy Fat 1 Grain	380

Fast breakfast idea	Category	Calories
<u>Peanut Butter Banana Waffle</u>: 1 Kashi waffle 1 small banana, sliced 1 tbsp peanut butter 8 oz. skim milk *Spread peanut butter on waffle and top with sliced banana.*	1 Grain 1 Fruit 1 oz. Meat & Beans; 2 tsp Healthy Fat 1 Milk	360
8 oz. plain low-fat Greek yogurt ½ cup blueberries ¼ cup granola ½ oz. almonds 1 tbsp Agave nectar	1 Milk ½ Fruit 1 Grain 1 oz. Meat & Beans; 1½ tsp Healthy Fat Extra (60)	395
16 oz. Green Machine Naked Juice 1 hard-boiled egg	2 Fruit/Vegetable 1 oz. Meat & Beans	360
<u>Breakfast sandwich</u>: 1 soy breakfast patty 1 slice Swiss cheese 1 Hearty Grains Whole Wheat English Muffin 1 medium pear	1 oz. Meat & Beans ½ Milk 2 Grains 1 Fruit	400

5-minute dorm-room lunches and dinners for 1

Pita Pocket Tuna *(420 calories)*
**Great pre-test meal*

3 oz. low-sodium light tuna in water	3 oz. Meat & Beans
1 tbsp olive-oil mayo	Extra (50 calories)
1 large whole-wheat pita	2 Grains
14 baby carrots	1 Vegetable
1 small apple, sliced	1 Fruit

Instructions:
1. Drain tuna and mix with mayo
2. Carefully separate pita and stuff with tuna mixture
3. Serve with sliced apple and carrots on the side.

Chunky Dorm-Room Chicken Soup *(455 calories)*

1 container (4.4 oz.) Minute Ready to Serve Brown Rice prepared according to package; use only half	1 Grain
½ cup (3 oz.) cooked chicken breast, diced (Tyson Grilled & Ready Oven Roasted Diced Chicken Breast)	3 oz. Meat & Beans
1 cup low- or reduced-sodium chicken broth	Extra (no calories)
1 cup frozen mixed vegetables	1 Vegetable
Small cluster of grapes (about 1 cup)	1 Fruit
5 Triscuit crackers	1 Grain

Instructions:
1. Combine broth and vegetables in a microwave-safe bowl and microwave on high for 3 minutes
2. Heat chicken on microwave-safe plate according to package directions
3. Combine all ingredients in a bowl and serve hot
4. Serve with cluster of grapes and crackers on the side

Chunky Dorm-Room "Chicken" Soup *(485 calories)*
(For vegetarians)

1 container (4.4 oz.) Minute Ready to Serve Brown Rice prepared according to package directions; use only half	1 Grain
12 Morningstar Farms Meal Starters Chik'n Strips	3 oz. Meat & Beans
1 cup low-sodium vegetable broth	Extra (no calories)
1 cup frozen mixed vegetables	1 Vegetable
Small cluster of grapes (about 1 cup)	1 Fruit
5 Triscuit crackers	1 Grain

Instructions:
1. Combine broth and vegetables in a microwave-safe bowl and microwave on high for 3 minutes.
2. Heat Chik'n Strips on microwave-safe plate according to package directions and dice into small pieces.
3. Combine all ingredients in a bowl and serve hot
4. Serve with cluster of grapes and crackers on the side

P.B. & Banana Flax Sandwich *(600 calories)*

2 slices whole-grain bread	2 Grains
2 tbsp peanut butter	2 oz. Meat & Beans; 4 tsp Healthy Fat
1 small banana	1 Fruit
8 oz. skim milk	1 Milk
1 tbsp ground flaxseed	½ oz. Meat & Beans; ¾ tsp Healthy Fat

Instructions:
1. Assemble peanut butter sandwich as usual but layer one side with banana slices and sprinkle with flaxseed before closing.

Mediterranean "Chicken" Wrap *(485 calories)*

1 6" whole-grain tortilla	1 Grain
2 tbsp hummus	1 oz. Meat & Beans
6 Morningstar Farms Meal Starters Chik'n Strips heated in microwave according to package directions	1½ oz. Meat & Beans
2 cups fresh spinach	1 Vegetable
¼ cup cranberry raisins	½ Fruit
¼ cup mandarin oranges, drained	¼ Fruit
2 tbsp shredded mozzarella cheese	1/3 Milk
2 tbsp balsamic vinaigrette salad dressing	2 tsp Healthy Fat

Instructions:
1. Heat tortilla in microwave for 15 seconds between two damp paper towels.
2. Spread hummus on tortilla; line Chik'n Strips in middle and roll up
3. Top spinach with raisins, mandarin oranges and cheese. Drizzle with salad dressing.

Crunchy 2-Bean Salad *(520 calories)*

¼ cup canned kidney beans, rinsed and drained	1 oz. Meat & Beans
½ cup frozen soybeans (edamame)	2 oz. Meat & Beans
½ cup sliced green bell pepper	½ Vegetable
½ cup diced tomatoes	½ Vegetable
2 tbsp Italian or balsamic vinaigrette dressing	2 tsp Healthy Fat
5 Triscuit crackers	1 Grain
1 cup unsweetened applesauce	1 Fruit

Instructions:
1. Cook soybeans in microwave-safe bowl according to package directions.
2. Combine kidney beans, soybeans, bell pepper and tomatoes and toss with dressing.
3. Top crackers with bean mixture

Nutty Pita Pocket "Burger" *(540 calories)*
**Great pre-test meal

1 Morningstar Garden Veggie Patty	2 oz. Meat & Beans
2 tbsp hummus	1 oz. Meat & Beans
1 cup fresh spinach	½ Vegetable
½ oz. walnuts	1 oz. Meat & Beans; 1½ tsp Healthy Fat
1 large whole-wheat pita	2 Grains
14 baby carrots	1 Vegetable
1 small apple, sliced	1 Fruit

Instructions:
1. Heat patty on microwave-safe plate according to package directions and slice into strips
2. Carefully separate pita and spread hummus on inside
3. Stuff pita with spinach, walnuts and patty strips and serve with sliced apple and carrots on the side.

Easy Tortilla Pizza (460 calories)	
Recipe submitted by Keisha, Gustavus Adolphus College	
1 6" whole-grain tortilla	1 Grain
¼ cup pizza sauce	Extra (30 calories)
¼ cup shredded cheese	¾ Milk
2 cup mixture of chopped broccoli, cauliflower, peppers, onions and carrots	2 Vegetables
½ cup kidney beans, rinsed and drained	2 oz. Meat & Beans
1 tsp olive oil (to sauté vegetables)	1 tsp Healthy Fat

Instructions:

1. Saute vegetables in olive oil and mix in beans until heated
2. Place tortilla in a pan on stove over medium heat. Top with sauce, vegetables, beans and cheese and heat until the cheese melts.

Sample meal plan and food-tracking sheet

Next, you'll see how everything comes together in a one-day sample meal plan. Once you know where each food fits, it's simple to plan healthy and energizing meals. Just follow the Power Meal Plates™ and you're on your way!

It helps to log your food once in a while, especially when you find yourself getting off track. It can be a real wake-up call to see it written down on paper and might even surprise you. The Food Tracking Sheet below allows you to write down what you eat and what food category it belongs in. This one is filled out using the foods in the one-day sample meal plan, but you can find a blank one in the appendix.

1-Day Sample Meal Plan

Meal	Menu	Category	Calories
Breakfast	1 cup cooked oats 1 cup strawberries 1 hard-boiled egg 1 tsp brown sugar	2 Grains (WG) 1 Fruit 1 oz. Meat & Beans Extra (15 calories)	300
Snack	6 oz. low-fat Greek yogurt ½ oz. walnuts♥ 1 tbsp agave nectar 16 oz. water	¾ Milk 1 oz. Meat & Beans; 1½ tsp Healthy Fat Extra (60 calories) 16 oz. water	225
Lunch	8 oz. skim milk 5 Triscuit crackers 2 cups fresh spinach 1 cup chopped cauliflower 2 oz. grilled chicken strips 3 tbsp Italian dressing 1 small apple 16 oz. water	1 Milk 1 Grain (WG) 1 Vegetable 1 Vegetable 2 oz. Meat & Beans 3 tsp Healthy Fat 1 Fruit 16 oz. water	525
Snack	1 oz. whole-grain cereal (Cheerios) 4 oz. skim milk	1 Grain (WG) ½ Milk	145
Dinner	1 cup brown rice with 2 cups steamed broccoli 3 tbsp shredded Cheddar cheese 3 oz. grilled salmon♥ 2 tsp canola oil♥♥ 1 tsp light-sodium soy sauce 2 Hershey's Dark Chocolate Kisses 16 oz. water	2 Grains (WG) 2 Vegetables ½ Milk 3 oz. Meat & Beans 2 tsp Healthy Fat Extra (no calories) Extra (50 calories) 16 oz. water	685
Snack	1 Kashi Oatmeal Dark Chocolate cookie 4 oz. skim milk	Extra (130 calories) ½ Milk	175
Totals:		Grains = 6 oz. (all WG) Meat & Beans = 7 oz. Milk = 3.25 cups Fruit = 2 cups Vegetables = 4 cups Healthy Fat = 6.5 tsp Omega 3-rich foods = 4 Water = 48 oz. Extras = 255 calories	2,055

Food-Tracking Sheet

Meal	Menu	Meat/ Beans (oz.)	Grains (oz.)	Milk (cups)
Breakfast	1 cup cooked oats 1 cup strawberries 1 hard-boiled egg 1 tsp brown sugar	1	2 WG	
Snack	6 oz. low-fat Greek yogurt ½ oz. walnuts♥ 1 tbsp agave nectar 16 oz. water	1		¾
Lunch	8 oz. skim milk 5 Triscuit crackers 2 cups fresh spinach 1 cup chopped cauliflower 2 oz. grilled chicken strips 3 tbsp Italian dressing 1 small apple 16 oz. water	2	1 WG	1
Snack	1 oz. whole-grain cereal (Cheerios) 4 oz. skim milk		1 WG	½
Dinner	1 cup brown rice with 2 cups steamed broccoli 3 tbsp shredded Cheddar cheese 3 oz. grilled salmon♥ 2 tsp canola oil♥♥ 1 tsp light-sodium soy sauce 2 Hershey's Dark Chocolate Kisses 16 oz. water	3	2 WG	½
Snack	1 Kashi Oatmeal Dark Chocolate cookie 4 oz. skim milk			½
Totals:		7 oz.	6 oz. (all WG)	3.25 cups

Fruit (cups)	Vegetables (cups)	Healthy Fat (tsp)	Omega 3's ♥	Water (oz.)	Extras (Calories)
1					15
		1½	♥	16	60
1	2	3		16	
	2	2	♥ ♥ ♥	16	50
					130
2 cups	4 cups	6.5 tsp	4 servings	48 oz.	255 calories

PLAN YOUR PLATE POWER HABITS™!

✓ Visit the Web site www.mayoclinic.com/health/calorie-calculator/nu00598 to determine how many calories your body requires to stay at its current weight.

✓ Eat breakfast every day, and be sure to include an ounce of protein.

✓ Choose the "better" or "best" option at lunch or dinner today.

✓ Get a feel for what a portion is supposed to look like by comparing all the foods you eat today with the standard portion sizes listed in the Food Lists. Are they larger, smaller or about the right size?

✓ Use the Power Meal Plates™ as a guide to plan one of your meals today.

✓ Fill half your lunch and dinner plates with colorful vegetables like broccoli.

✓ Eat healthy and energizing snacks between meals to keep your energy up.

✓ Write your own Plan Your Plate Power Habit™: _____

_____

_____

The Bottom Line

You don't have to be perfect! Even if you choose the "better" option instead of the "best," it's better for you than the original. Start by being more conscious of what you're eating. Next, pay attention to portion sizes. Remember, your bagel should be the size of a hockey puck, not the size of a DVD. Choose a Plan Your Plate Power Habit™ from the list above to practice today, or get creative and make up your own. Don't forget to record it on your Power Habit™ Tracking Chart in the back of the book!

Secret 18

GRADE-A SHOPPING

What's in it for you?

✓ Take the guesswork out of healthy grocery shopping

✓ Save money on your grocery bill

✓ Learn the best foods to put in your cart in each aisle

✓ Avoid the two grocery aisles that will drain your brain

✓ Find out what the must-have foods are for your dorm or apartment

If you get into the habit of eating from a vending machine, you're going to start looking like one.

College is probably the first time in your life you're having to grocery-shop on your own. You can go about this one of two ways: Grab a cart and just start filling it mindlessly with foods that are cheap, easy to prepare and not so good for you; or load it with foods that fit within your tight budget, are healthy and simple to prepare and won't make you pile on the pounds. If it's in your dorm or apartment, you'll eat it! Start by making some good choices when you shop—choices that will make a positive impact on your body and grades.

At first I dreaded going to the grocery store, but once I knew what to buy, it was much easier to eat healthy! I always make sure my dorm is stocked with peanut butter, yogurt, popcorn, dried fruit, nuts, granola bars and, of course, soup!

—KEN, freshman at the University of Florida

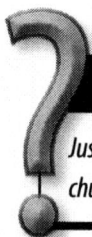

DID YOU KNOW?

Just by shopping only the perimeter of the grocery store, you can eliminate a huge chunk of many unhealthy, highly processed foods!

6 money-saving tips:

1. Shop from a list and stick to it!

The only way to eat a balanced diet is to shop for one. When preparing your list, think "food groups" rather than just "food." Which groups are missing from your dorm room or kitchen—fruits, vegetables, grains, milk, meat and beans or healthy fats? If you eat most of your meals in a dining hall, you'll still want to have some food in your dorm in case you have to miss a meal. The grocery list in the appendix will help you choose the best possible foods in each aisle.

2. Don't shop when you're hungry.

This spells danger! You'll load your cart with more junk food and less of the foods your body needs to stay healthy and energized. Eat a small meal or snack before you head to the store.

3. Use your rewards card.

Most grocery stores have rewards cards you can sign up for to receive discounts. They're free, so take advantage. Some stores even offer savings on gas when you use your rewards card.

4. *Use coupons!*

You don't have to buy a Sunday newspaper and clip coupons like your Mom. Here are three Web sites that offer printable coupons. They change every week, so be sure to check them frequently. This can really add up to big savings!

✓ www.coolsavings.com

✓ www.coupons.com

✓ www.couponsurfer.com

5. *Beware of pre-made foods.*

You'll definitely pay for the convenience of visiting the prepared-foods department of the grocery store.

6. *Swap one version of a food for another and save money!*

Instead of this:	Buy this:
Small individual containers of yogurt	Large tub of yogurt
Single-serving snack-pack foods (100-calorie packs)	Full-size bag (portion it out in sandwich bags)
Pre-cut vegetables and prepackaged lettuce	Baby carrots, cherry tomatoes and other fresh veggies (cut them yourself)
Instant-oatmeal packs	Large tub of Quaker Oatmeal (it takes only 1½ minutes to cook in a microwave)
Fresh fruits and vegetables	Frozen fruits and vegetables
Name brand	Store brand
Bottled juice	Frozen concentrate

Navigate the aisles like a health nut

All grocery stores are set up pretty much the same way. You'll want to spend 75% of your time shopping the outer aisles and 25% in the inner aisles. The inner aisles have more of the salty, sugary and fatty processed foods. The foods on the perimeter of the store are fresher and more nutritious overall.

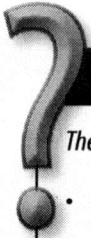

Outer Aisles:

Produce:

Fruits and vegetables are the most nutrient-packed foods in the grocery store. They have only one ingredient—the food itself! Always reach for the produce that's in season to save money (you'll know by the price).

Dairy:

If you don't have trouble digesting them, low-fat milk and yogurt should be staples in your refrigerator. Choose 1% or skim milk and watch out for added sugars in the yogurt. Most have some, so pick the one with the least amount if possible. When selecting cheeses, stay away from processed cheeses like Cheese Whiz, American cheese and Laughing Cow and go for hard natural cheeses like cheddar, mozzarella, Swiss, Parmesan and soft cheeses like cottage cheese.

Eggs:

Eggs have the highest-quality protein of any food, containing all nine essential amino acids. If you don't have a stove, stop by the salad bar and pick up seven hard-boiled eggs for the week and eat one every day for a snack.

Frozen foods:

Depending on what you select, these could be your best friend or your worst enemy. Frozen vegetables, fruits and beans are nutrition powerhouses. They're picked at peak freshness and quickly frozen, so they hold on to their nutrients. Some are even more nutritious than fresh produce! As fresh fruits and vegetables travel to your grocery store and sit in their bins waiting to be purchased, light and oxygen start breaking down the nutrients.

Watch out for frozen vegetables and fruits with added salt and sugar. To get the best nutritional buy, look for those without added sauces or syrups. Many frozen dinners are loaded with sodium. If you must buy them, try to find the reduced-sodium versions.

Fresh-meat department:

Fresh meat is always a better option than the deli counter. Deli meats have gone through processing and contain a load of sodium. Take a look at the difference in sodium between fresh turkey and turkey lunch meat:

3 ounces of fresh turkey = 25.6 grams of protein, 44 mg of sodium

3 ounces of deli turkey = 14.5 grams of protein, 863 mg of sodium

Bakery department:

Who can resist the aroma of fresh-baked cookies, cakes and doughnuts when passing through the bakery department? Hidden in this department is one of the most delicious discoveries in the store. No, not the chocolate chip cookies the size of your hand—the fresh-baked bread! For the most nutrition for your grocery dollar, pick the whole-grain varieties. These breads freeze well, too, so if you don't eat the whole loaf within a few days, drop it in a freezer bag and store in your freezer.

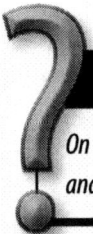

DID YOU KNOW?

On average, organic foods contain slightly higher levels of trace minerals, vitamin C and antioxidants than conventionally grown crops but are generally more expensive.

Inner Aisles:

Juice aisle:

Though 100% fruit and vegetable juices are nutritious and will fulfill your fruit and vegetable requirements, fresh and frozen are always best. Not only do you get more fiber, but they do a better job of keeping you full. Try drinking 8 ounces of apple juice for your morning snack and then eat a large apple with the skin on for your afternoon snack. The whole apple takes longer to digest, so you'll feel full longer. If you decide to buy juice, look for 100% fruit juice and low-sodium vegetable juices.

Cereal aisle:

This is the most versatile aisle in the store. Having so many different cereals to choose from can be overwhelming. Don't panic! Check for the following when making your selection:

✓ Whole grain: The first term on the ingredient panel should be "whole grain", "whole oat" or "whole wheat"

✓ Grams of fiber: The more fiber the better

✓ Grams of sugar: One teaspoon of sugar equals 4 grams, so when you're reading the food label on your favorite box of cereal, picture the teaspoons of sugar adding up. For example, one serving of Kellogg's Corn Pops has 12 grams of sugar. That's like swallowing 3 teaspoons of white sugar!

✓ Grams of saturated fat: Look for those with the least amount of saturated fat

✓ Grams of trans fat: Choose those with no grams of trans fat per serving and no partially hydrogenated oils on the food label.

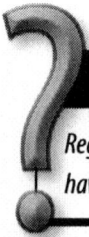

DID YOU KNOW?

Regular and instant oatmeal are both considered whole grains. Instant oatmeal can have up to 200 mg of sodium per packet, but regular oatmeal contains no sodium.

Instant hot cereals like oatmeal and Cream of Wheat can be very nutritious choices for breakfast, much better than a glazed doughnut. Two things to keep in mind are cost and sodium. You're going to pay more because they're packaged in individual servings. For about the same price, you'll get 30 servings out of a canister of oatmeal and only eight if you opt for the instant cereal. Regular oatmeal is just as convenient, can be prepared in 90 seconds in your microwave and has no sodium. Compare that with upwards of 200 mg of sodium in a packet of instant hot cereal.

Granola bars are a college student's best friend and are typically found in the cereal aisle. The same rules apply when selecting a granola bar as with cereal. Look for those that are whole grain, higher in fiber and lower in sugar, saturated fat and trans fat. Just because it's a granola bar doesn't mean it's good for you!

Snack-food aisle:

Crackers, pretzels, potato chips, nuts and tortilla chips can be found here. Watch out because you'll also find extra sodium, saturated fat and trans fat if you're not careful.

Many tortilla chips now come in whole-grain varieties, so if you're going to buy snack foods, these are the best ones. Unsalted or lightly salted nuts are a good nutritional buy, too! Popcorn is a whole grain and can be a wonderful snack. Notice the words *can be*. Some brands of microwave popcorn are loaded with butter, trans fats and saturated fat. In these cases, you'd be better off eating potato chips! Be a label reader and choose snacks that are trans fat-free.

Crackers should be whole-grain. Ritz Crackers and Saltines aren't whole-grain, but Triscuits, Wheat Thins and Kashi crackers are.

Cookie and snack-cake aisle:

Trans fat can hide out in this aisle, especially in the crème-filled cookies and cakes. Certain types of cookies that you may think are a healthier option can contain trans fats, such as some varieties of fig cookies, vanilla wafers, graham crackers and animal crackers.

Cupcakes, mini-doughnuts, muffins and other types of snack cakes might seem like a good buy at first glance. They can be cheap, but what you save in dollars you'll lose in energy. These treats are typically high in sugar, total and saturated fat and possibly trans fats. Some have as many as 7 teaspoons of sugar, 5 grams of saturated fat and 2 grams of trans fat per serving. If you want a sharp brain, skip the snack-cake aisle altogether.

Beverage and soft-drink aisle:

It's okay to enjoy a soda once in a while; just be sure to put it into perspective. Each 12-ounce can has 150 calories and 10 teaspoons of sugar. Because they're empty calories, they offer zero nutrition for your "calorie dollar." Think of soft drinks more like a dessert—you don't order a hot fudge ice cream sundae after every meal, do you? Some healthier alternatives to soda are:

✓ Flavored water without artificial sweeteners (e.g., Hint Water)

✓ Sparkling flavored waters (e.g., La Croix)

✓ Bottled water

✓ True Lemon packets (add to water for a refreshing lemon flavor without added calories or artificial sweeteners)

Canned and dried food aisles:

These can make your life much easier. Most canned foods are filled with sodium, however, so be a health-conscious label reader. Some canned products, like soups, tuna fish and vegetables, offer a lower-sodium or "no added salt" alternative. Aim for these when possible, and always rinse vegetables and beans in cold water to slash the sodium even further.

Pasta sauce can either be creamy (alfredo) or tomato-based (marinara). Stick with tomato-based to save on calories and saturated fat. A half-cup of alfredo sauce has 200 calories and 18 grams of fat (10 grams saturated), while a half-cup of marinara has 80 calories and 4.5 grams of fat (0.5-gram saturated).

Condiments and oils:

A little goes a long way with condiments. Salad dressings, soy sauce, mayonnaise, oils, barbecue sauce, ketchup, mustard, pickles and olives are all considered condiments. Watch out, because these innocent little fixings can turn a healthy meal into one that's high in sodium, calories and fat.

Olive oil-based mayonnaise is a better choice than traditional mayo. With half the calories and fat, a third of the saturated fat and virtually no cholesterol, olive-oil mayonnaise is just as creamy as the "real" thing!

If you use only a couple of tablespoons of salad dressing, there really is no need to go fat-free. Choose oil-based salad dressings like Italian and balsamic vinaigrette over creamy ones like blue cheese and ranch. Creamier dressings can be higher in saturated fat and don't spread as easily, which means you'll end up using twice as much.

Candy and other sweets:

Candy is a non-nutritive food, meaning it offers calories, sugar and sometimes fat, without much nutrition. Dark chocolate is the exception, because it's loaded with antioxidants, those powerful substances that protect your body against certain diseases such as cancer and heart disease. If you're going to indulge in something sweet, make it dark chocolate. The bitterness you taste is actually the antioxidants. The higher the percentage of cacao, the darker the chocolate and the more antioxidants it contains. Studies have also shown that dark chocolate increases blood flow to the brain, helping you stay sharp and focused. An added bonus to eating dark chocolate is you don't need much of it to satisfy your sweet tooth. You could probably pop six milk chocolate candies into your mouth and still crave more, but when you switch to dark, you'll need only one or two.

Dry pasta and other grains:

There's a wealth of opportunity here to work some whole grains into your diet. Remember, your target is at least three servings of whole grains every day. Choose whole-grain pasta, barley, brown rice and, if you're in the mood for something adventurous, quinoa or whole-grain couscous. Unless you buy these from a bulk bin, they can be more costly.

Boxed dinners and canned pasta:

There are two aisles in the grocery store you should skip altogether: the snack-cake aisle and this aisle. Cheesy instant potatoes and spaghetti in a can are convenient to have on hand when you're looking for a quick meal, but you won't feel much like studying afterward. You can just as easily microwave some brown Minute Rice and frozen vegetables and mix in a half-cup of canned black beans. See *Secret 17: Plan Your Plate* for more quick and easy meal ideas.

Your first trip to the grocery store is always the longest. Take your time, explore the store and know where the healthiest foods are located and your shopping trips will be a piece of cake. Don't forget to check out the handy Grade-A Grocery List in the appendix.

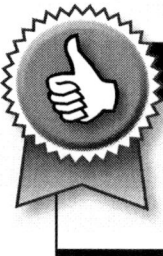

GOOD IDEA!

Always have some healthy staple foods in your dorm or apartment. It makes healthy snacking so much easier, and you don't have to rely on the vending machine!

Must-have foods for your dorm or kitchen

1. *Smart Balance Smart 'n Healthy Popcorn*
2. *Brown instant rice* (e.g., Minute Rice Ready to Serve Brown Rice or Uncle Ben's)
3. *Canned beans:* pinto, kidney, black, black-eyed peas, etc.
4. *Canned soup with 50% less sodium* (Campbell's Healthy Request, Progresso 50% Less Sodium)

5. **Chicken** *(e.g., Tyson Grilled & Ready Chicken Breast Strips, Fillets, or Oven Roasted Diced Chicken Breast)*

6. **Kashi Oatmeal Dark Chocolate Cookies**

7. **Dark chocolate**

8. **Dried fruit:** *apricots, figs, prunes, raisins*

9. **Flintstone Vitamins**

10. **Fruit:** *apples, bananas, berries, pears, oranges, etc.*

11. **Green-tea bags**

12. **Hummus**

13. **Mayonnaise** *(olive oil-based)*

14. **Veggie burgers**

15. **Nuts: peanuts, walnuts, almonds**

16. **Oatmeal** *(e.g., Quaker Oatmeal in canister)*

17. **Peanut Butter** *(e.g., Smucker's Natural Peanut Butter)*

18. **Pouched light tuna fish, salmon or chicken** *(e.g., Tyson Premium Chunk Chicken Breast)*

19. **Salad dressing, non-creamy** *(e.g., Italian or balsamic vinaigrette)*

20. **Skim milk or low-fat soy milk**

21. **Soybeans** *(frozen)*

22. **String cheese**

23. **Vegetables:** *carrots, bell peppers, broccoli, cauliflower, cherry tomatoes, spinach, etc.*

24. **V8 Juice** *(low-sodium)*

25. **Whole-grain cereal** *(e.g., Kashi, Cheerios, low-fat granola, Frosted Mini-Wheats)*

26. **Whole-grain cereal bars** *(e.g., Kashi, Nature Valley Crunchy Granola Bars)*

27. **Whole-grain crackers** *(e.g., Triscuit Hint of Salt, Kashi Crackers)*

28. **Whole-grain tortilla chips** *(e.g., Garden of Eatin' Blue Chips)*

29. **Whole-wheat bread**

30. **Yogurt** *(choose those with the least amount of sugar, such as low-fat plain or vanilla Greek yogurt)*

Best vending-machine picks

Although you'd do best to prepare, there will be times when you're faced with an empty stomach and the only food in sight is behind the glass in a vending machine. Don't freak out—you can actually find at least one or two decent options in most vending machines. Here are your best bets:

- ✓ Granola bars: Nature Valley or Kashi
- ✓ Nuts or seeds
- ✓ Baked! Lays
- ✓ Sun Chips
- ✓ Pretzels
- ✓ Dried fruit
- ✓ Bottled water
- ✓ Yogurt
- ✓ Smartfood popcorn
- ✓ Mini rice cakes

GRADE-A SHOPPING POWER HABITS™!

✓ Always shop from a list! Use the Grade-A Grocery List in the appendix and highlight the foods you plan to buy.

✓ Load your cart with healthy proteins and carbohydrates so that you'll always have good food available for a quick snack.

✓ Limit junk food to one purchase.

✓ Since you're probably sharing a refrigerator, limit your perishable food items to milk, yogurt, cheese, fresh fruits and vegetables, veggie burgers and frozen vegetables.

✓ Put a stop to impulse purchases—eat something before you shop.

✓ Kashi products are your best friends. Look for Kashi granola bars, cereal, cookies and crackers.

✓ Read the food label before putting it in your cart.

✓ Write your own Grade-A Shopping Power Habit™: _____

_____

_____

The Bottom Line

If it's in your dorm or apartment, you'll eat it. Take care of your body—be proactive and fill your grocery cart with smart, health-conscious foods. Your budget will be tight, so it's important to make your food choices work for you rather than against you. Choose the Grade-A Shopping Power Habits™ that are comfortable for you and hit the grocery store! Don't forget to record it on your Power Habit™ Tracking Chart in the back of the book!

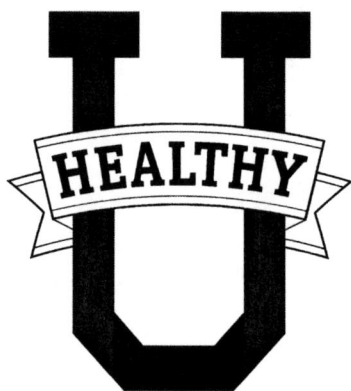

Secret 19

FINDING HEALTHY
FAST FOOD

What's in it for you?

✓ Take the guesswork out of ordering the healthiest
foods at your favorite restaurants

✓ Cut your calories in half

✓ Don't compromise taste

*You control what you order at a restaurant—
the menu doesn't control you!*

Restaurant food doesn't have to be bad for you. You can find at least
one healthy option on every menu; you just have to know what
to look for. The tables below show you the healthiest menu items at
the most well-known fast-food restaurants. They also provide tips on
your best bets at Chinese, Italian and steakhouse restaurants. Whether
it's lunch, dinner or feeding your 3 a.m. munchies, you'll be prepared the
next time you set foot into a restaurant or cruise through a drive-thru.

Arby's

Best Options	Calories	Carbs	Protein	Fat
Regular Roast Beef	360	37	22	14
Arby's Melt	390	39	22	16
Ham & Swiss Melt	300	37	18	8
Roast Chicken Sandwich	400	40	24	16
Chopped Farmhouse Salad—Turkey & Ham with half the balsamic vinaigrette dressing	315	12.5	23	20
Chopped Farmhouse Salad—Roast Chicken with half the balsamic vinaigrette dressing	315	13.5	23	19
Chopped side salad with half the balsamic vinaigrette dressing	135	6.5	4	11
Junior Roast Beef	210	24	12	8
Junior Ham & Cheddar Sandwich	210	26	13	6
1% Chocolate Milk	160	28	8	2

When you don't want to compromise: *With the Beef & Cheddar, instead of a Large Beef & Cheddar with a large order of Curly Fries, order a regular Beef & Cheddar with a small order of Potato Cakes and save 680 calories and 38 fat grams.*

Burger King

Best Options	Calories	Carbs	Protein	Fat
Hamburger	260	27	13	10
Cheeseburger	300	28	16	14
Tendergrill Chicken Sandwich with lettuce and tomato	360	40	55	7
BK Veggie Burger with lettuce, tomato and ketchup	310	40	22	7
Fresh Apple Fries with Caramel Sauce	70	16	0	0.5
Tendergrill Chicken Garden Salad with half dressing (Ken's Light Italian)	290	11.5	34	13.5
Garden Salad with half dressing (Ken's Light Italian)	130	9.5	4	9.5
Kids Breakfast Muffin Sandwich	210	23	9	8
1% low-fat chocolate milk (8 oz.)	180	31	2.5	9

Best Options	Calories	Carbs	Protein	Fat
Fat-free milk (8 oz.)	100	14	10	0
Minute Maid Apple Juice (6.67 oz.)	100	23	0	0
Minute Maid Orange Juice (10 oz.)	140	33	2	0
Late-night option				
Whopper Junior (with no mayo)	260	29	13	10

When you don't want to compromise: *With the Whopper, order the Whopper Junior and **save 410 calories and 30 fat grams.***

DID YOU KNOW?

The amount of fat in a Burger King Whopper is equivalent to a half-stick of butter.

DID YOU KNOW?

Just by exchanging the larger order of fries for a side salad, you'll save 410 calories and 18 grams of fat.

Chipotle

Best Options	Calories	Carbs	Protein	Fat
Vegetarian Fajita Burrito Bowl: rice, black beans, fajita vegetables, tomato salsa, lettuce and half the cheese	345	54	15	17.5
Chicken Fajita Burrito Bowl: chicken, rice, black or pinto beans, fajita vegetables, tomato salsa, lettuce and half the cheese	535	55	55	24.5
Salad of lettuce, black beans, fajita vegetables, tomato salsa, chicken and half the Chipotle Honey Vinaigrette salad dressing and half the cheese	510	34	44	25

When you don't want to compromise: *With the steak burrito, instead of the steak fajita burrito, order a steak fajita burrito with half the cheese, half the rice and no sour cream and **save 235 calories and 16 fat grams.***

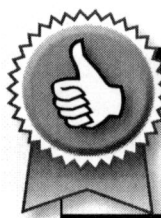

GOOD IDEA!

When you order off of Chipotle's kid's menu, you get the same food but the portion sizes are smaller and it's cheaper—BONUS!

KFC

Best Options	Calories	Carbs	Protein	Fat
Original Chicken Breast with no skin or breading	160	2	31	3.5
Grilled Chicken Breast	210	0	34	8
KFC Grilled Fillet	140	1	26	3
KFC Snacker, Honey BBQ	210	32	13	3
Honey BBQ Sandwich	320	47	24	3.5
Doublicious with Grilled Fillet with no sauce	340	32	35	8
Grilled Chicken Caesar Salad with Marzetti Light Italian Dressing and no croutons	235	8	33	7.5
Caesar Side Salad with Marzetti Light Italian Dressing and no croutons	55	4	3	2.5
Grilled Chicken BLT Salad with Marzetti Light Italian Dressing	245	10	35	8.5
House Side Salad with Marzetti Light Italian Dressing	30	5	1	.5
Green Beans	20	3	1	0
Mashed Potatoes with gravy	120	19	2	4
Corn on the Cob (3")	70	16	2	.5
BBQ Baked Beans	210	41	8	1.5
Sweet Kernel Corn	100	21	3	0.5
Sargento Light String Cheese	50	1	6	2.5

When you don't want to compromise: With the breaded chicken breast, instead of the Extra Crispy Chicken Breast & Mashed Potatoes with Gravy and a Biscuit, order the Original Chicken Breast, Mashed Potatoes with Gravy and Baked Beans and **save 120 calories and 26.5 fat grams.**

Long John Silver's

Best Options	Calories	Carbs	Protein	Fat
Grilled Pacific Salmon	150	2	24	5
Grilled Tilapia	110	1	22	2.5
Freshside Grille Smart Choice Salmon	280	27	27	7
Freshside Grille Smart Choice Tilapia	250	27	25	4.5
Freshside Grille Smart Choice Shrimp Scampi	330	29	20	15
Corn Cobbette without butter	90	14	3	3
Hushpuppy (1)	60	9	1	2.5
Breadstick	170	29	6	3.5
Vegetable Medley	50	8	1	2
Rice	180	37	4	1

When you don't want to compromise: *With the fish sandwich, instead of the Ultimate Fish Sandwich with Coleslaw & Fries, order a Fish Sandwich with Corn Cobbette and Vegetable Medley and **save 290 calories and 17 fat grams.***

McDonald's

Best Options	Calories	Carbs	Protein	Fat
Egg McMuffin	300	30	18	12
English muffin	160	27	5	3
Hotcakes (no syrup or margarine)	350	60	8	9
Hotcakes (1 syrup, 1 pat margarine)	570	105	8	13.5
Fruit & Maple Oatmeal	290	57	5	4.5
Snack-size fruit and walnut salad	210	31	4	8
Fruit 'n Yogurt Parfait	160	31	4	2
Hamburger	250	31	12	9
Cheeseburger	300	33	15	12
Honey Mustard Snack Wrap	260	27	18	9
Premium Grilled Chicken Classic Sandwich	420	51	32	10

McDonald's — Best Options	Calories	Carbs	Protein	Fat
Chipotle BBQ Snack Wrap	260	28	18	9
Small order of french fries	230	29	3	11
Premium Southwest Salad with grilled chicken	320	30	30	9
Side salad	20	4	1	0
Low-fat balsamic vinaigrette salad dressing	40	4	0	3
Low-fat Italian salad dressing	60	8	1	2.5
Ice cream cone	150	24	4	3.5
Oatmeal raisin cookie	150	22	2	6
Apple dippers with low-fat caramel dip	100	23	0	0.5
Strawberry Banana Smoothie (12 oz.)	210	49	2	0.5
Wild Berry Smoothie (12 oz.)	210	48	2	0.5
1% low-fat milk	100	12	8	2.5
1% low-fat chocolate milk	170	26	9	3
Minute Maid apple juice box	100	23	0	0
Orange juice (small)	150	30	2	0
Coffee with 1 cream	20	0	0	2
Nonfat cappuccino (small)	60	9	6	0
Nonfat latte (small)	90	13	9	0
Iced nonfat latte (small)	50	7	5	0

When you don't want to compromise: With the Double Cheeseburger, order a side salad with Italian dressing or a Fruit & Yogurt Parfait instead of the large order of french fries and a bottled water instead of a large Coke and **save 650 calories and 23 fat grams.**

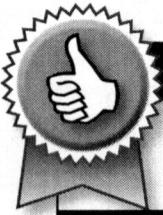

GOOD IDEA!

If you're looking for a fun way to control your calories at McDonald's— order a Happy Meal! Most have less than 600 calories

Papa John's Pizza

Best Options	Calories	Carbs	Protein	Fat
1 slice small Garden Fresh Pizza (original crust)	140	20	5	4.5
1 slice small Hawaiian BBQ Chicken Pizza (original crust)	240	31	10	8
1 slice small Cheese Pizza (original crust)	180	25	7	6
2 Breadsticks with 1 container pizza sauce for dipping	310	57	8	5.5

When you don't want to compromise: *If you order the pepperoni, ham and sausage pizza, eat only one slice and blot the grease with a napkin and* ***save 230 calories and 9 fat grams.***

I was very involved in undergraduate student government at Ohio State, which, given its size, was like being in the government of a small country. I learned early on that free pizza was literally the grease that kept the machine (the student body) moving. I theorized one week that I could dine only on free pizza offered at clubs, organizations, associations, rallies and the like. I began on a Monday during fall quarter and did not pay for pizza or any food, for that matter, until the following Sunday morning. It was as disgusting as it was wonderful.

—PETER, Graduate of Ohio State University

Panera

Best Options	Calories	Carbs	Protein	Fat
Breakfast & Breads				
Egg & Cheese on Ciabatta	390	43	19	15
Breakfast Power Sandwich	340	31	23	14
Strawberry Granola Parfait	310	44	9	11
Whole Grain Baguette	140	29	6	1
Whole Grain Bagel	340	67	13	2.5

Panera — Best Options	Calories	Carbs	Protein	Fat
Sandwiches (To make it even better, ask for whole-grain bread)				
Half Tomato & Mozzarella on Ciabatta	380	48	15	15
Half Turkey Artichoke on Focaccia	370	43	21	13
Half Asiago Roast Beef on Asiago Cheese	350	32	24	14
Half Mediterranean Veggie on Tomato Basil	300	49	11	7
Half Napa Almond Chicken Salad on Sesame Semolina	340	45	15	13
Half Tuna Salad on Honey Wheat	240	32	9	8
Half Mediterranean Veggie on Tomato Basil	300	50	11	7
Half Smoked Ham & Swiss on Stone-Milled Rye	290	32	22	8
Half Smoked Turkey Breast on Country	210	33	16	1.5
Salads (Ask for dressing on the side and use only half; Balsamic Vinaigrette or Greek Herb Vinaigrette are your best choices)				
Full Asian Sesame Chicken	410	31	31	20
Full BBQ Chopped Chicken with Balsamic Vinaigrette Dressing	480	51	31	20
Thai Chopped Chicken Salad	390	36	34	15
Full Classic Café	170	18	2	11
Fruit Cup	60	16	1	0
Soups				
Low Fat Chicken Tortilla	190	24	10	6
Low Fat Garden Vegetable with Pesto	160	28	5	3.5
Low-Fat Chicken Noodle	140	23	5	3
Low-Fat Vegetarian Black Bean	170	29	10	4
Drinks				
Low Fat Black Cherry Smoothie—16 oz.	290	63	6	1.5
Low Fat Mango Smoothie-16 oz.	230	51	6	1.5
Low Fat Strawberry Smoothie w/Ginseng—16 oz.	260	59	6	1.5

Best Options	Calories	Carbs	Protein	Fat
Low Fat Wild Berry Smoothie—16 oz.	290	67	6	1.5
Iced Green Tea—16 oz.	90	23	0	0
Cafe Latte—8.5 oz.	120	11	8	4.5
Cappuccino—8.5 oz.	120	11	8	4.5
Chai Tea Latte—10 oz.	200	32	7	4.5
Coffee (black)—12 oz.	0	0	0	0
Orange Juice-small (8 oz.)	110	26	2	0
Apple Juice—8 oz.	120	29	0	0

When you don't want to compromise: *With the Italian Combo on Ciabatta, order a Half Italian Combo and a Half Garden Vegetable Soup and* **save 380 calories and 18 fat grams.**

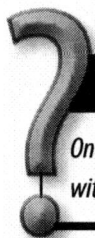

DID YOU KNOW?

One bagel at Panera counts as four servings of grains! How about splitting it with a friend?

Starbucks

Best Options	Calories	Carbs	Protein	Fat
Chocolate Vivanno Smoothie with skim milk	250	48	18	2
Orange Mango Vivanno Smoothie with skim milk	260	51	15	2
Strawberry Vivanno	280	56	15	1.5
Iced coffee with skim milk—grande	30	4	3	0
Brewed coffee	5	0	0	0
Brewed Tazo tea	0	0	0	0
Non-fat Latte—grande	130	19	13	0
Non-fat Cappuccino—grande	80	12	8	0
Iced Non-fat Caffe Latte —grande	90	13	8	0
Coffee Frappuccino Light Blended Beverage—grande	110	27	3	0

Starbuck's — Best Options	Calories	Carbs	Protein	Fat
Non-fat Flavored Steamed Milk—grande	200	37	12	0
Non-fat Tazo Awake Tea Latte –grande	160	32	8	0
Tazo Iced Tea—unsweetened	0	0	0	0
Dark Cherry Yogurt Parfait	310	61	10	4
Strawberry & Blueberry Yogurt Parfait	300	60	7	3.5
Reduced-Fat Turkey Bacon with Egg Whites on English Muffin	320	43	18	7
Egg White Spinach & Feta Wrap	280	33	18	10
Reduced-fat Turkey Bacon with Egg White on English Muffin	340	47	22	10
Perfect Oatmeal	140	25	5	2.5
Perfect Oatmeal with nut-medley topping	240	27	7	11.5
Deluxe Fruit Blend	90	23	0	0
Protein Artisan Snack Plate	370	36	13	19
Farmer's Market Salad	230	24	8	12
Picnic Pasta Salad	320	53	16	5
Chicken on Flatbread with Hummus Artisan Snack Plate	250	27	17	9
Roasted Vegetable Panini	350	48	13	12
Turkey & Swiss Sandwich	390	36	34	13
Tarragon Chicken Salad Sandwich	420	46	32	13

When you don't want to compromise: With the Caffé Mocha, order a tall Caffé Mocha with no whipped cream and **save 240 calories and 15 fat grams.**

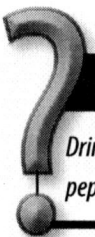

DID YOU KNOW?

Drinking a Venti Caffé Mocha from Starbucks is like eating two slices of pepperoni pizza.

Subway

Best Options	Calories	Carbs	Protein	Fat
Breakfast				
Egg White & Cheese Muffin Melt	150	24	12	3.5
Egg White & Cheese (with ham) Muffin Melt	170	24	14	4
Egg White & Cheese Mornin' Flatbread	170	21	9	5
Egg White & Cheese (with ham) Mornin' Flatbread	180	22	12	5
Subs with 6 Grams of Fat or Less*				
6" Ham	290	46	18	4.5
6" Oven Roasted Chicken	320	47	23	5
6" Roast Beef	320	45	24	5
6" Subway Club	310	46	23	4.5
6" Sweet Onion Chicken Teriyaki	380	59	26	4.5
6" Turkey Breast	280	46	18	3.5
6" Turkey Breast and Ham	280	46	18	4
6" Veggie Delite	230	44	8	2.5
Flatbread Sandwiches				
6" Veggie Delite	240	42	8	4.5
6" Black Forest Ham	300	44	17	7
6" Roast Beef	330	43	23	7
6" Roasted Chicken Breast	330	45	22	7
6" Subway Club	320	44	22	7
6" Sweet Onion Chicken Teriyaki	390	57	25	7
6" Turkey Breast & Ham	290	44	17	6
6" Turkey Breast	290	44	17	6
Soups				
Chicken Tortilla	110	11	6	1.5
Chipotle Chicken Corn Chowder	140	22	6	3

Subway — Best Options	Calories	Carbs	Protein	Fat
Soups *continued*				
Fire-Roasted Tomato	130	24	6	1
Minestrone	90	17	4	1
Roasted Chicken Noodle	80	12	6	2
Rosemary Chicken and Dumpling	90	14	6	1.5
Spanish Style Chicken with Rice	110	16	6	2.5
Tomato Garden Vegetable with Rotini	90	20	3	0.5
Vegetable Beef	100	17	5	2
Salads with 6 Grams of Fat or Less**				
Ham	110	11	12	3
Oven Roasted Chicken	130	9	19	2.5
Roast Beef	140	10	18	3.5
Subway Club	140	11	17	3.5
Sweet Onion Chicken Teriyaki	200	24	20	3
Turkey Breast	110	11	12	2
Turkey Breast & Ham	120	11	12	2.5
Veggie Delite	50	9	3	1
Grilled Chicken & Baby Spinach	130	10	20	2.5

*Subs with 6 grams of fat or less include nine-grain wheat bread, lettuce, tomato, onion, green pepper and cheese.
**Salads do not include salad dressing or croutons.

When you don't want to compromise: *With the Meatball Marinara Sub, order it with Baked Lays and bottled water instead of with Doritos and a large sweet tea and **save 430 calories.***

Taco Bell

Best Options	Calories	Carbs	Protein	Fat
Chicken Burrito Supreme	400	51	21	12
Steak Burrito Supreme	390	51	17	13
Bean Burrito	370	55	14	10

Best Options	Calories	Carbs	Protein	Fat
Fresco Bean Burrito	350	57	12	8
Fresco Burrito Supreme- Chicken	350	50	18	8
Fresco Burrito Supreme- Steak	340	50	15	8
Fresco Chicken Soft Taco	150	18	12	3.5
Fresco Crunchy Taco	150	13	7	7
Fresco Grilled Steak Soft Taco	150	19	9	4
Fresco Soft Taco	180	20	8	7
Gordito Nacho Cheese—Chicken	270	29	15	10
Gordito Nacho Cheese—Steak	260	29	12	11
Gordito Supreme— Chicken	270	29	17	10
Gordito Supreme— Steak	270	29	14	11
Mexican Rice	120	20	2	3.5
Pintos-n-Cheese	170	20	9	6
Chicken Soft Taco	190	20	13	6

*When you don't want to compromise: If you have a taste for nachos, instead of Volcano Nachos, order the Cheesy Nachos and **save 700 calories and 43 fat grams.***

Wendy's

Best Options	Calories	Carbs	Protein	Fat
Ultimate Chicken Grill Sandwich	360	42	33	7
Baked potato	270	61	7	0
Baked potato with small chili	480	82	24	6
Junior Hamburger	230	26	12	8
Junior Cheeseburger	270	27	15	11
Grilled Chicken Go Wrap	260	25	19	10
Junior Hamburger Patty (add to a side salad)	90	0	8	7
Ultimate Chicken Grill Fillet (add to a side salad)	120	1	26	1.5
Side salad	25	5	1	0

Wendy's — Best Options	Calories	Carbs	Protein	Fat
Side salad with Ultimate Chicken Grill Fillet and half-packet of Italian vinaigrette dressing	180	8	27	4.5
Side salad with Junior Hamburger patty and half-packet of Italian vinaigrette dressing	150	7	9	10
Mandarin Orange Cup	90	21	1	0
Apple Slices	40	9	0	0
TruMoo low-fat white milk	100	12	8	2.5
TruMoo low-fat chocolate milk	140	22	7	2.5
Small chocolate or vanilla Frosty	310	52	8	8

When you don't want to compromise: *If you have a taste for bacon on your burger, instead of a Double Baconator, order a Jr. Bacon Cheeseburger and **save 580 calories and 39 fat grams.***

Panda Express

Best Options	Calories	Carbs	Protein	Fat
Steamed Rice (8.1 oz.)	380	86	7	0
Mixed Veggies (side)	70	13	4	0.5
String Bean Chicken Breast	170	13	15	7
Broccoli Beef	130	13	10	4
Kobari Beef	210	20	15	7
Veggie Spring Roll	160	22	4	7
Egg Flower Soup	90	15	3	2
Hot & Sour Soup	100	12	4	3.5

When you don't want to compromise: *If you order the Sweet & Sour Chicken, get it with steamed rice instead of fried rice and **save 150 calories and 16 fat grams.***

Steakhouse (Outback)

Best Options	Calories	Carbs	Protein	Fat
Seared Ahi Tuna (small)	177	6	9	12
Outback Special—6 oz.	332	1	37	19

Best Options	Calories	Carbs	Protein	Fat
Grilled Chicken on the Barbie & Fresh Seasoned Veggies (both with no butter)	465	32	72	9
Teriyaki Marinated Sirloin (9 oz.)	418	17	57	12
Joey Sirloin	292	0	31	18
Atlantic Salmon with no butter	363	2	39	21
Lobster Tails with no butter	233	6	47	2
Roasted Filet Sandwich	814	88	55	26
Roasted Filet Sandwich—share half with a friend	407	44	27.5	13
Fresh Steamed Green Beans with no butter	46	9	0	0
Fresh Seasonal Veggies with no butter	50	10	2.5	0.5
Sweet Potato with no butter	420	92	5.5	4
Potato Boats	165	32	4	2
Baked Potato with cheese only	357	65	10	7
House Salad with Tangy Tomato Salad Dressing and three grilled shrimp	435	37	20.5	23.5

When you don't want to compromise: *If you order the Sirloin steak, get it with a House Salad with Tangy Tomato Dressing and Fresh Seasoned Veggies instead of the Classic Blue Cheese Wedge Salad and Fries and* **save 588 calories and 34 fat grams.**

Italian Food (Olive Garden)

Best Options	Calories	Carbs	Protein	Fat
Bruschetta	610	100	26	13
Bruschetta split with a friend	305	50	13	6.5
1 Breadstick	150	28	4	2
Pasta e Fagioli	130	17	10	2.5
Minestrone Soup	100	18	2.5	1
Zuppa Toscana	170	24	10.5	4
Garden Fresh Salad (ask for half the amount of dressing)	235	19.5	5	15
Capellini Pomodoro	840	141	31	17

Olive Garden — Best Options	Calories	Carbs	Protein	Fat
Capellini Pomodoro split with a friend	420	70.5	15.5	8.5
Linguine alla Marinara	430	76	17	6
Herb-Grilled Salmon	510	5	64	26
Shrimp Primavera	730	110	45.5	12
Shrimp Primavera split with a friend	365	55	22.75	6
Venetian Apricot Chicken	380	32	54	4
Steak Toscano	590	62	40.5	20

When you don't want to compromise: *If you order the Spaghetti & Meatballs, split it with a friend and order Minestrone Soup instead of breadsticks and* ***save 605 calories and 26 fat grams.***

A note on Chinese food

Although the staples of this cuisine are rice and vegetables, not all Chinese food is healthy. Use the tips below to help you make wiser choices.

Healthy Tips for Chinese Carryout

✓ Use chopsticks! You'll eat more slowly and take in less oil that way.

✓ Skip the sauce, or ask for half if you must have it. Thick sauces and gravies are made from sugar and flour or cornstarch and add a lot of extra calories. Instead, choose hot mustard sauce, oyster sauce or hoisin sauce. Most are high in sodium, so use them sparingly, and ask for low-sodium sauces when possible.

✓ Ask for more vegetables and less meat. You're probably used to ordering it the other way around. You'll still get plenty of meat and fewer calories.

✓ For more nutrients and fiber, always ask for brown rice instead of white. Remember, brown rice is a whole grain.

✓ Ask for your meal to be prepared in vegetable stock instead of beef or chicken stock to save on fat and calories.

✓ Choose the lighter option when possible:

Instead of this:	Order this:	
Appetizer: Fried Egg Rolls Spare Ribs	**Appetizer:** Egg Drop Soup Hot & Sour Soup	Wonton Soup Spring Roll
Battered, deep-fried dishes: General Tso's Chicken Sweet & Sour Pork Fried Tofu	**Stir-fried dishes:** Chop Suey Chow Mein Tofu	Moo Goo Gai Pan Shrimp with Garlic Sauce
Fried Rice or White Rice	Brown Rice	
Fried Dumplings	Steamed Dumplings	

Treat your fork like a fork, not a shovel

A note on buffet-dining

All-you-can-eat buffets can seem like a dream come true when you're on a tight budget. The secret is to use them wisely. Treat buffets like regular restaurants where you order from a menu. To stop the dream from becoming a fat nightmare, promise yourself you won't make more than two or three trips to the buffet:

✓ **Before you grab a plate,** walk around the buffet and scope out the food just like you'd browse a menu before ordering. Look for the salad bar, hot vegetables, lean proteins and grains/starchy vegetables that aren't swimming in pools of cheese sauce or butter.

✓ **Trip One:** Start with a broth-based soup or spinach salad with non-creamy dressing. For your drink, try a tall glass of ice water with a lemon or lime wedge or skim milk. Don't be tempted by the ever-flowing fountain-drink, lemonade or fruit-punch machine. All they offer are empty calories—a whopping 200 calories or more per glass!

✓ **Trip Two:** Select your entrée. Fill your plate with a hefty dose of vegetables, a quarter lean protein, and a quarter whole-grain roll, pasta, rice or starchy vegetable

✓ **Trip Three** (only if you aren't already full): If you feel like treating yourself to a dessert, choose the one (not the five) that looks most appealing to you. An oatmeal cookie, angel food cake with fresh berries, frozen yogurt topped with fruit or just plain fruit salad will always be the smarter choices.

HEALTHY FAST FOOD POWER HABITS™!

✓ Since restaurant portions are often huge, split the meal with a friend and save on calories and money or ask for a doggie bag!

✓ Opt for grilled, baked, stir-fried, broiled, roasted or steamed instead of fried, deep-fried, crispy, battered, creamy or sautéed.

✓ Ask for non-creamy dressing for your salad (on the side), and use only half.

✓ Just say no to supersized meals.

✓ Choose fish and skinless poultry over beef and pork.

✓ Order your favorite coffee drink with skim or 1% milk.

✓ Ask for whole-wheat bread or pasta and brown rice instead of white.

✓ Skip the heavy sauces and gravies.

✓ Ask for a side of veggies instead of french fries.

✓ Treat beverages just like food and don't overdrink. Choose water or skim milk. If you must have a soda, limit it to one and ask for lots of ice.

✓ Write your own Healthy Fast Food Power Habit™: _____

_____

_____

The Bottom Line

Dining out can be enjoyable and healthy. Once you're used to choosing the better menu option, over time you'll come to prefer it. The next time you dine away from your dorm, dining hall or apartment, pick a Healthy Fast Food Power Habit™ from above and commit to it or create your own. Don't forget to record it on your Power Habit™ Tracking Chart in the back of the book!

Secret 20
(Elective)

VEGETARIAN 101

What's in it for you?

✓ Go meatless without worrying about nutrition

✓ Love meat? Learn how to be a flexible vegetarian

✓ Keep your calories in check

Just because you're a vegetarian doesn't automatically qualify you as a healthy eater

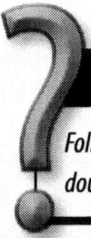

DID YOU KNOW?

Following a vegetarian diet can be unhealthy if you're not careful. Doughnuts and double-fudge brownies are both meatless, after all!

Contrary to popular belief, following a vegetarian diet:

✓ Won't cause you to be malnourished, as long as it's well-balanced

✓ Doesn't mean eating tree bark, foods that taste like tree bark, or only fruits and vegetables

✓ Isn't always healthy

Choosing a vegetarian lifestyle is becoming more and more popular these days, especially among college students. The good news is that more vegetarian food products are being made available at your local grocery store. Even better news: They're convenient, affordable and tasty.

Just because you're a vegetarian doesn't automatically qualify you as a healthy eater. Plenty of college students consider themselves to be vegetarian but live on sweets and potato chips. If planned correctly, it can be a nutritious diet. If you're a vegetarian or are considering this option, you'll want to pay close attention to this Secret.

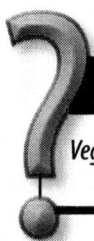

DID YOU KNOW?

Vegetarians aren't necessarily thinner than meat-eaters.

As a vegetarian, I always struggled to find veg-friendly options in the dining hall. I sought solace in Chicago's many vegan and vegetarian eateries and microwaveable Morningstar Farms fake chicken nuggets. The culmination of my indulgence in vegetarian goodness came when a fellow intern (who is vegan) and I obtained a press pass to attend the Green Festival held at Navy Pier. While we did sit in on two lectures, including one on the power of green algae, we spent the majority of the day sampling everything from four varieties of rice to organic milk to Luna bars to chips and salsa and veggie burgers. In some cases, we went back for thirds! The memory I have is not one of heartburn but one of laughter. We are still friends and we still try to re-create that experience with free samples from Whole Foods, but sadly, it's not the same.

—ALYSSE, graduate of Loyola University

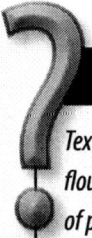

DID YOU KNOW?

Textured vegetable protein (TVP) is a dehydrated meat substitute made from soy flour. To prepare it, simply rehydrate with water or vegetable broth. It's a great source of protein for vegetarian students and can be used as a substitute for ground beef. Bob's Red Mill is one brand of TVP found in most grocery stores.

5 types of vegetarians:

1. The Vegan:

Vegans eat no animal products whatsoever. Meat, poultry, seafood, dairy products, eggs and any products made from these foods are all excluded.

2. The Lacto-Vegetarian:

Lacto-vegetarians eat dairy products such as milk, yogurt, cheese and butter but exclude meat, poultry, seafood, eggs and any products made from these foods.

3. The Ovo-Vegetarian:

Ovo-vegetarians eat eggs but exclude meat, poultry, seafood, dairy products and any products made from these foods.

4. The Lacto-Ovo-Vegetarian:

Lacto-ovo-vegetarians eat eggs and dairy products but exclude meat, poultry, seafood and any products made from these foods.

5. The Flexitarian:

Flexitarians are flexible vegetarians, or people who eat mostly a plant-based diet and occasional meat, poultry or fish. This might be a good option for you if you've tried to follow a vegetarian lifestyle but missed the taste of meat.

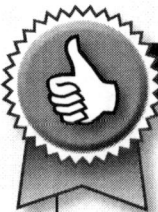

GOOD IDEA!

If you're thinking about trying a vegetarian lifestyle, instead of giving up meat "cold turkey," try easing into it. For the first two weeks, go meatless three days a week. For the next two weeks, bump it up to five days a week. At the end of the month, tack on another two days and you're there!

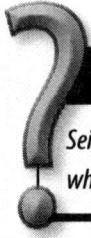

6 nutrients vegetarians need to focus on:

1. Calcium:

Dairy products are the richest sources of calcium, an essential mineral for strong bones and teeth. Because they eliminate dairy products, vegans and ovo-vegetarians are especially at risk for a calcium deficiency if they don't substitute appropriately. To be sure you aren't missing out on this important mineral, take a look at the table below for non-animal sources of calcium.

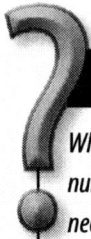

2. Iron:

Your red blood cells depend on dietary iron. It's a key mineral involved in energy metabolism and a healthy immune system. The most usable form of iron is called heme iron and comes from animal products like meat, poultry and seafood. Plant sources of iron are considered non-heme and are not as readily absorbed. Foods rich in vitamin C, like tomatoes and oranges, help your body absorb iron. The next time you sit down with a plate of iron-rich beans, try mixing in some diced tomatoes and red peppers for better iron absorption.

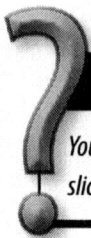

3. **Protein:**

   Protein is important for healthy skin, muscles and organs. Most people name this nutrient as the one lacking in vegetarian diets. Actually, non-meat sources of protein such as soy, legumes, lentils, nuts, seeds and whole grains contain enough protein for a well-balanced diet.

4. **Vitamin D:**

   Found in dairy products, fortified cereals, margarine, fish, eggs and sunlight, vitamin D is often lacking in vegetarian and non-vegetarian diets alike. Vitamin D aids in the absorption of calcium and plays a role in bone health.

5. **Vitamin B12:**

   This vitamin helps form your red blood cells, maintain a healthy nervous system and build your DNA. It's found only in animal products and in some fortified cereals and soy products. If you're a vegan, it can be very difficult for you to get enough vitamin B12, so you should consider taking a daily multivitamin.

6. **Zinc:**

   Just like iron, zinc is more easily absorbed when it comes from animal products as opposed to plants. Plant sources of zinc include whole grains, soy, legumes, nuts and wheat germ. Zinc is important for wound-healing and a healthy immune system.

Nutrient	Vegetarian Food Sources:	
Calcium	-Blackstrap molasses -Calcium-fortified cereals -Calcium-fortified juices -Calcium-fortified soy, almond, or rice milk -Calcium-set tofu -Cow's milk (if lacto- or lacto-ovo-vegetarian) -Dairy products: soy or cow cheese, milk, yogurt -Green leafy vegetables: bok choy, Chinese cabbage, collards, kale, okra, spinach, turnip greens -Soybeans	
Iron (combine with vitamin C-rich foods to increase absorption)	-Beans -Dried fruit -Enriched breads and cereals -Leafy green vegetables -Nuts -Soybeans and tofu -Tomato juice -Whole-wheat bread and other whole grains	Vitamin C- rich foods: -Melons -Citrus fruits -Pineapple -Strawberries -Kiwi -Broccoli -Peppers -Tomatoes

Nutrient	Vegetarian Food Sources:
Protein	-Beans -Dairy products -Grains -Peanut butter and nuts -Soy milk -Tofu -Veggie burger or other meat substitutes
Vitamin D	-Cow's milk -Egg yolk -Fortified cereals -Fortified orange juice -Fortified soy milk
Vitamin B-12	-Cow's milk -Eggs -Fortified breakfast cereals -Some brands of nutritional yeast (such as Red Star Vegetarian Support Formula) -Some brands of soy milk
Zinc	-Beans (including soybeans) -Nuts and seeds -Nut and seed butters -Wheat germ -Whole grains (some fortified refined grains)

Vegetarian meal planning

Healthy U makes it easy for vegetarians to eat well-balanced meals both on campus and off. The Food Lists in *Secret 17: Plan Your Plate* include non-animal sources of protein, iron, calcium, zinc, vitamin D and vitamin B-12. The breakfast and lunch/dinner Power Meal Plates™ are built with the vegetarian student in mind, too; simply choose the vegetarian option in each food list (marked by either a for "vegetarian" or ▼ for "vegan").

1-Day Sample Meal Plan for Vegetarians

Meal	Menu	Category	Calories
Breakfast	1 cup cooked oats 1 cup strawberries 1 hard-boiled egg or soy sausage patty 1 tsp brown sugar	2 Grains (WG) 1 Fruit 1 oz. Meat & Beans Extra (15 calories)	300
Snack	6 oz. low-fat Greek or soy yogurt ½ oz. walnuts♥ 1 tbsp agave nectar 16 oz. water	¾ Milk 1 oz. Meat & Beans; 1 ½ tsp Healthy Fat Extra (60 calories) 16 oz. water	225
Lunch	8 oz. skim, soy, almond or rice milk 5 Triscuit crackers 2 cups fresh spinach 1 cup chopped cauliflower 3 tbsp shredded cheddar cheese/soy cheese 8 Morningstar Farms Meal Starters Chik'n Strips 3 tbsp Italian dressing 1 small apple 16 oz. water	1 Milk 1 Grain (WG) 1 Vegetable 1 Vegetable ½ Milk 2 oz. Meat & Beans 3 tsp Healthy Fat 1 Fruit 16 oz. water	600
Snack	1 oz. whole-grain cereal (Cheerios) 4 oz. skim, soy, rice or almond milk	1 Grain (WG) ½ Milk	145
Dinner	1 cup brown rice with 2 cups steamed broccoli 1/3 cup extra-firm tofu♥ 2 tsp canola oil♥♥ 1 tsp light-sodium soy sauce 2 Hershey's Dark Chocolate Kisses 16 oz. water	2 Grains (WG) 2 Vegetables 3 oz. Meat & Beans 2 tsp Healthy Fat Extra (no calories) Extra (50 calories) 16 oz. water	525
Snack	1 Kashi Oatmeal Dark Chocolate cookie 4 oz. skim, soy, rice or almond milk	Extra (130 calories) ½ Milk	175
Totals:		Whole Grain = 6 oz. Meat & Beans = 7 oz. Milk = 3.25 cups Fruit = 2 cups Vegetables = 4 cups Healthy Fat = 6.5 tsp Omega 3-rich foods = 4 Water = 48 oz. Extras = 255 calories	1970

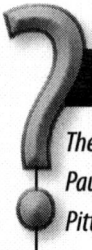

DID YOU KNOW?

The following celebrities are vegetarians: Hayden Panettiere, Alicia Silverstone, Paul McCartney, Gwyneth Paltrow, Moby, Ellen DeGeneres, Woody Harrelson, Brad Pitt and Pink.

Vegetarian food suppliers:

Here's a list of food suppliers offering vegetarian and vegan options broken down by category. If you're looking for a certain vegetarian product, ask the grocer to order it for you.

Meat Substitutes:

Boca: *BocaBurger.com*
Burgers, beef crumbles, chicken patties, chicken nuggets

Fantastic Foods: *FantasticFoods.com*
Falafel, tofu scrambles, burger crumbles

Gardenburger: *Gardenburger.com*
Burgers, chicken patties

Lightlife Foods: *Lightlife.com*
Deli slices, bacon, hot dogs, ground beef

MorningStar Farms: *Morningstarfarms.com*
Burgers, chicken patties, hot dogs, ribs, chicken strips, chicken nuggets, ground beef

Tofurky: *Tofurky.com*
Deli slices, hot dogs, tofurky (vegetarian turkey)

Yves Veggie Cuisine: *YvesVeggie.com*
Breakfast links, sausage, deli slices, hot dogs

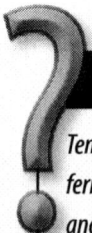

DID YOU KNOW?

Tempeh (pronounced "TEM pay") is a traditional Indonesian food made from cooked fermented soybeans that are formed into chunky yet tender "cakes." Tempeh is another great meat substitute, packing in about 21 grams of protein in 4 ounces.

Dairy Alternatives:

Eden Foods: *EdenFoods.com*
Soy milk, grains, sea vegetables

Nasoya: *Nasoya.com*
Soy milk, mayonnaise, tofu, dressings

Silk: *SilkSoyMilk.com*
Soy milk, creamer, yogurt

Tofutti: *Tofutti.com*
Ice cream, soy cheese, cream cheese, sour cream

Westsoy: *Westsoy.biz*
Soy milk, rice milk

Egg Replacements:

Ener-G Foods: *Ener-G.com*
Egg replacer

General:

Amy's Kitchen: *Amys.com*
Prepared and frozen foods

Dixie USA: *Dixiediner.com*
Wide variety of vegan products

Westbrae Natural: *Westbrae.com*
Beans, pasta, condiments

Salad Dressings:

Annie's Naturals: *AnniesNaturals.com*
Salad dressings

VEGETARIAN POWER HABITS™!

✓ If you're a vegan, be sure to get plenty of calcium. Three cups (8 ounces) of low-fat calcium-fortified soy, rice or almond milk each day will do the trick.

✓ Take a daily multivitamin and calcium supplement with added vitamin D, especially if you think you aren't regularly eating vegetarian sources of calcium, iron, vitamin D, vitamin B-12 and zinc.

✓ Don't shy away from certain menu items like grilled chicken salad or spaghetti and meatballs just because they have meat in them. Ask for the dish anyway, but without the meat. If the restaurant serves beans, lentils or veggie burgers, request that your meal be topped with one of those instead.

✓ Eat a bowl of fortified cereal like Total every day.

✓ To stay satisfied, eat a serving of protein such as tofu or beans at each meal.

✓ Combine plant sources of iron with vitamin C for best absorption. For example: black beans and rice with diced tomatoes.

✓ Be sure to eat one to two servings of walnuts, soybeans and other vegetarian sources of omega 3 fatty acids every day.

✓ Write your own Vegetarian Power Habit™: _____

_____

The Bottom Line

A vegetarian isn't much different from a meat-eater. You still have to be mindful of what you're eating and follow a well-balanced diet because there are plenty of non-meat choices that are far from healthy! If you're a vegetarian or are thinking of dabbling in the vegetarian lifestyle, choose the Vegetarian Power Habit™ you're most comfortable with and put it into action today. Don't forget to record it on your Power Habit™ Tracking Chart in the back of the book!

Secret 21
(Required Reading)

DON'T IGNORE
AN EATING DISORDER!

What's in it for you?

✓ Save your own life (or someone else's!)

*Whether it's for you or a friend, please seek help
if you suspect an eating disorder*

If you think you or someone you know has an eating disorder, please don't ignore it. Seek help, even if you aren't 100% sure.

Common forms of eating disorders include anorexia nervosa, bulimia nervosa and binge-eating disorder. Below is an explanation of each from the National Eating Disorders Association.

DID YOU KNOW?

In a survey of women on a college campus, 91% had attempted to control their weight through dieting, and 22% dieted "often" or "always" (Kurth et al., 1995).

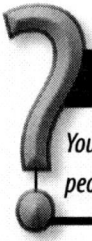

? DID YOU KNOW?

You can't tell if a person has an eating disorder simply by looking at him or her. Many people affected by an eating disorder actually have a normal body weight.

Anorexia nervosa

Anorexia nervosa is characterized by self-starvation and excessive weight loss.

Symptoms include:

✓ Refusal to maintain body weight at or above a minimally normal weight for height, body type, age and activity level

✓ Intense fear of weight gain or being "fat"

✓ Feeling fat or overweight despite dramatic weight loss

✓ Loss of menstrual periods

✓ Extreme concern with body weight and shape

Health consequences:

✓ Reduction of bone density (osteoporosis), resulting in brittle bones

✓ Severe dehydration, which can result in kidney failure

✓ Fainting, fatigue and overall weakness

✓ Dry hair and skin; hair loss is common

✓ Abnormally slow heart rate and low blood pressure, increasing the risk of heart failure

Signs that someone you know may have anorexia nervosa:

✓ Dramatic weight loss

✓ Dresses in layers to hide weight loss

✓ Is preoccupied with weight, food, calories, fat grams and dieting

✓ Refuses to eat certain foods, progressing to restrictions against whole categories of food (e.g., no carbohydrates)

✓ Makes frequent comments about feeling "fat" or overweight despite weight loss

✓ Complains of constipation, abdominal pain, cold intolerance, lethargy and excess energy

✓ Denies feeling hungry

✓ Develops food rituals (e.g., eating foods in certain orders, excessive chewing, rearranging food on a plate)

✓ Cooks meals for others without eating

✓ Consistently makes excuses to avoid mealtimes or situations involving food

✓ Maintains an excessive, rigid exercise regimen despite weather, fatigue, illness, or injury, citing the need to "burn off" calories taken in

✓ Withdraws from usual friends and activities and becomes more isolated, withdrawn, and secretive

✓ Seems concerned about eating in public

✓ Resists maintaining body weight at or above a minimally normal weight for age and height

✓ Has intense fear of weight gain or being fat even though he or she is underweight

✓ Has disturbed experience of body weight or shape, undue influence of weight or shape on self-evaluation, or denial of the seriousness of low body weight

✓ Post-puberty female loses menstrual period

✓ Feels ineffective

✓ Has strong need for control

✓ Exhibits inflexible thinking

✓ Has overly restrained initiative and emotional expression

Bulimia nervosa

Bulimia nervosa is characterized by a secretive cycle of binge eating followed by purging (vomiting). It includes eating extraordinarily large amounts of food in one meal and then getting rid of the food through vomiting, laxative abuse or overexercising.

Symptoms include:

- ✓ Repeated episodes of binging and purging
- ✓ Feeling out of control during a binge and eating beyond the point of comfortable fullness
- ✓ Purging after a binge (typically by self-induced vomiting, abuse of laxatives, diet pills or diuretics, excessive exercise or fasting)
- ✓ Frequent dieting
- ✓ Extreme concern with body weight and shape

Health consequences:

- ✓ Electrolyte imbalances that can lead to irregular heartbeats and possibly heart failure and death
- ✓ Inflammation and possible rupture of the esophagus from frequent vomiting
- ✓ Tooth decay and staining from stomach acids released during frequent vomiting
- ✓ Chronic irregular bowel movements and constipation as a result of laxative abuse
- ✓ Potential for gastric rupture during periods of binging

Signs that someone you know may have bulimia nervosa:

- ✓ In general, behaviors and attitudes indicate that weight loss, dieting, and control of food are becoming primary concerns
- ✓ Evidence of binge eating, including disappearance of large amounts of food in short periods of time or presence of empty wrappers and containers indicating consumption of large amounts of food

✓ Evidence of purging behaviors, including frequent trips to the bathroom after meals, signs or odors of vomiting, presence of wrappers or packages of laxatives or diuretics

✓ Appears uncomfortable eating around others

✓ Develops food rituals (e.g., eats only a particular food or food group such as condiments, excessive chewing, doesn't allow foods to touch)

✓ Skips meals or takes small portions of food at regular meals

✓ Steals or hoards food in strange places

✓ Drinks excessive amounts of water

✓ Uses excessive amounts of mouthwash, mints and gum

✓ Hides body with baggy clothes

✓ Maintains excessive, rigid exercise regimen despite weather, fatigue, illness, or injury, citing the need to "burn off" calories

✓ Shows unusual swelling of the cheeks or jaw area

✓ Has calluses on the back of the hands and knuckles from self-induced vomiting

✓ Teeth are discolored, stained

✓ Creates lifestyle schedules or rituals to make time for binge-and-purge sessions

✓ Withdraws from usual friends and activities

✓ Looks bloated from fluid retention

✓ Frequently diets

✓ Shows extreme concern with body weight and shape

✓ Has secret recurring episodes of binge eating (eating in a single period of time an amount of food that's much larger than most people would eat under similar circumstances), feels lack of control over ability to stop eating

✓ Purges after a binge (e.g., self-induced vomiting, abuse of laxatives, diet pills or diuretics, excessive exercise, fasting)

✓ Body weight is typically within the normal weight range; may be overweight

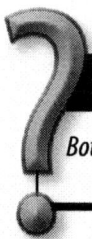

? DID YOU KNOW?

Both females and males are susceptible to eating disorders.

Binge-eating disorder (also known as compulsive overeating):

Binge-eating disorder is characterized primarily by periods of un-controlled, impulsive or continuous eating beyond the point of feeling comfortably full. While there is no purging, there may be sporadic fasts or repetitive diets and often feelings of shame or self-hatred after a binge. People who overeat compulsively may struggle with anxiety, depression and loneliness, which can contribute to their unhealthy episodes of binge eating. Body weight may vary from normal to mild, moderate or severe obesity.

Health consequences:

- ✓ High blood pressure
- ✓ High cholesterol levels
- ✓ Heart disease as a result of elevated triglyceride levels
- ✓ Type 2 diabetes
- ✓ Gallbladder disease

Signs that someone you know may have binge-eating disorder:

- ✓ Disappearance of large amounts of food in short periods of time or presence of empty wrappers and containers indicating consumption of large amounts of food
- ✓ Develops food rituals (e.g., eats only a particular food or food group such as condiments, excessive chewing, doesn't allow foods to touch)
- ✓ Steals or hoards food in strange places
- ✓ Hides body with baggy clothes
- ✓ Creates lifestyle schedules or rituals to make time for binging sessions
- ✓ Skips meals or takes small portions of food at regular meals
- ✓ Has periods of uncontrolled, impulsive or continuous eating beyond the point of feeling comfortably full

✓ Does not purge

✓ Engages in sporadic fasting or repetitive dieting

✓ Body weight varies from normal to mild, moderate or severe obesity

What's my ideal body weight anyway?

You won't find your ideal body weight on a chart or a table. To find the weight that's right for you, you have to listen to your body. It's the weight that keeps you healthy, gives you energy and makes you strong. If you feel tired all the time, get sick often and feel weak, the way to find your ideal body weight is by:

✓ Eating balanced, nutritious meals

✓ Enjoying regular, moderate exercise

✓ Understanding that the not-so-nutritious foods have a place in your diet, too, but only a small place.

If you follow these simple steps, your body will naturally settle at its ideal weight.

Embrace your body

Embrace your body, because it's *your* body. Resist the urge to compare it with your friends' bodies or the bodies of the actors in your favorite television shows. A good way to start is by learning the keys to your ideal body.

The 6 Keys to Your Ideal Body:

🗝 Treat your body with respect

🗝 Fuel it with a variety of foods

🗝 Exercise moderately

🗝 Give it enough rest

🗝 Resist the pressure to judge yourself and others based on shape, weight or size

🗝 Eat what you want when you're truly hungry and stop when you're full

What should you say if you suspect your friend has an eating disorder?

1. Set aside a time for a private meeting with your friend to discuss your concerns openly and honestly in a caring, supportive way.

2. Communicate your concerns. Share your memories of specific times when you've been concerned about your friend's eating or exercise behaviors. Explain that you think these instances may indicate that there's a problem that needs professional attention.

3. Ask your friend to explore these concerns with a counselor, doctor, dietitian or other health professional who's knowledgeable about eating issues. If you feel comfortable doing so, offer to help your friend make an appointment or accompany your friend on the first visit.

4. If your friend refuses to acknowledge that there's a problem or any reason for you to be concerned, restate your feelings and the reasons for them and leave yourself open and available as a supportive listener.

5. Avoid placing shame, blame or guilt on your friend regarding his or her actions or attitudes.

6. Avoid suggesting simple solutions.

7. Express your continued support. Remind your friend that you care and want him or her to be healthy and happy.

Could you have an eating disorder?

The following 12 questions are from Eating Disorders Anonymous. This quiz is not meant to diagnose an eating disorder but can help to identify an otherwise-unforeseen problem. If you answer yes to three or more of these questions, you may have an eating disorder.

Can you relate?	Yes	No
Are you, at times, unable to stop (or start) eating even when you really want to?		
Do you feel guilty about eating?		
Are you, at times, afraid to eat?		
Do you feel as if people watch you when you eat?		
Do you sneak food or hoard food so people won't know how much or how little you're eating?		
Are you ritualistic about eating?		
Do you obsess about food or body weight?		
Do you spend much of your time thinking about what, when and where you'll eat next?		
Are you constantly making resolutions about eating and not following through?		
Do you often feel panicked?		
Do you regularly feel useless, unworthy, disgusted or powerless?		
Do you often eat so much or little that it affects your plans for the day?		
Total:		

Did you answer yes to three or more questions? If so, please seek help.

Where to turn to for help

Your campus health center is the place to start. You can feel comfortable opening up about a possible eating disorder here because the staff is specially trained to help you. All information you share with the health professional is kept confidential.

Another place to turn for help if you or someone you know is struggling with an eating disorder is the National Eating Disorders Association. The phone number for its information and referral help line is 1-800-931-2237

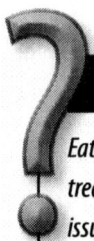

DID YOU KNOW?

Eating disorders are not a choice. They develop over time and require appropriate treatment to address the complex medical and psychiatric symptoms and underlying issues (Source: National Eating Disorders Association).

The Bottom Line

Whether it's for you or a friend, please seek help if you suspect an eating disorder. If you ignore an eating disorder, it won't go away—it will only get worse. And tragically, for some people it's fatal.

APPENDIX

Glossary

alpha-linolenic acid (ALA) - The only omega-3 fatty acid found in vegetable products; a fatty acid essential for health.

amino acid - A compound that serves as a building block of protein.

anorexia nervosa - A serious disorder in eating behavior that is characterized especially by a pathological fear of weight gain, leading to faulty eating patterns, malnutrition and usually excessive weight loss.

antioxidants - Substances that may protect your cells against the effects of free radicals.

artificial sweeteners - Sweeteners that do not contain appreciable calories.

B-vitamins- Vitamins that help your body convert food to energy and help form red blood cells.

baked - Cooked in an oven or oven-type appliance.

battered - Covered with a mixture of flour, eggs and milk before cooking.

béarnaise sauce – A sauce made with egg yolks and butter.

beta-carotene- A vitamin that acts as an antioxidant, protecting cells against oxidation damage. The body converts it to vitamin A.

binge-eating disorder (compulsive overeating)- An eating disorder characterized primarily by periods of uncontrolled, impulsive or continuous eating beyond the point of feeling comfortably full. While there is no purging, there may be sporadic fasts or repetitive diets and often feelings of shame or self-hatred after a binge. Body weight may vary from normal to mild, moderate or severe obesity.

braise - To cook meat or poultry over low heat in a covered utensil in a small amount of liquid or steam.

broil - To cook by direct heat on a rack.

bulimia nervosa - An eating disorder characterized by a secretive cycle of binge eating followed by purging (vomiting). It entails eating extraordinarily large amounts of food in one meal and then getting rid of the food through vomiting, laxative abuse or overexercising.

calcium - A mineral present in teeth and bones; it is required by the body to help muscles and blood vessels contract and expand, to secrete hormones and enzymes and to send messages through the nervous system.

caffeine - A bitter substance found in coffee, tea, soft drinks, chocolate, kola nuts and certain medicines. It has many effects on the body's metabolism, including stimulating the central nervous system.

carbohydrate - Any of various neutral compounds of carbon, hydrogen, and oxygen (as sugars, starches, and celluloses) most of which are formed by green plants and which constitute a major class of animal foods; contains 4 calories per gram.

chia seed - The seed of the Salvia hispanica (chia) plant.

cholesterol - A waxy, fatlike substance that occurs naturally in all parts of the body.

choline - A B-complex vitamin that is a constituent of lecithin.

coconut water - The clear liquid inside young coconuts.

complete protein - A protein source providing all the amino acids.

complex carbohydrates - Often referred to as "starchy" foods, they are carbohydrates that have three or more sugars and include legumes, starchy vegetables, whole-grain breads and cereals.

deep-fry - To cook food in enough hot fat for submersion or floating.

dehydration - Loss of water from the body that occurs when water output exceeds water input.

dietary fiber - The part of the plant that your body can't digest. It adds bulk to your diet and makes you feel full faster, helping you control your weight. Fiber helps digestion and helps prevent constipation.

docosahexaenoic acid (DHA)- An omega 3 fatty acid found in fish.

dopamine - A monoamine neurotransmitter found in the brain and essential for the normal functioning of the central nervous system.

eicosapentaenoic acid (EPA)- An omega 3 fatty acid found in fish.

electrolytes - Minerals in your body that have an electric charge. They are in your blood, urine and body fluids. Maintaining the right balance of electrolytes helps your body's blood chemistry, muscle action and other processes. Sodium, calcium, potassium, chlorine, phosphate and magnesium are all electrolytes. You get them from the foods you eat and the fluids you drink.

endorphin - A natural substance in the brain that has analgesic properties.

epinephrine (also known as adrenaline)- A hormone and neurotransmitter that increases heart rate, constricts blood vessels, dilates air passages and participates in the fight-or-flight response of the sympathetic nervous system.

essential amino acid - An amino acid that is essential to human health but cannot be manufactured in the body.

essential fatty acid - An unsaturated fatty acid that is essential to human health but cannot be manufactured in the body.

fat - A term referring either to the lipids in foods or to body fat, both of which are composed mostly of triglycerides; dietary fat contains 9 calories per gram.

flaxseed - The seed of the flax plant.

flexitarian - A flexible vegetarian, or a person who eats mostly a plant-based diet and occasional meat, poultry or fish.

free radicals - Molecules produced when your body breaks down food, or through environmental exposures to tobacco smoke, radiation, etc. Free radicals can damage cells and may play a role in heart disease, cancer and other diseases.

fry - To cook in fat.

hangover - The sum of unpleasant physiological effects that follow heavy consumption of alcoholic beverages.

hara hachi bu - The Okinawan practice of calorie control, which means "eat until you're 80% full."

high-density lipoprotein (HDL) – The lipoprotein that transports cholesterol from the tissues of the body to the liver so it can be gotten rid of (in the bile). (Lipoproteins are the form in which lipids are transported in the blood.) HDL cholesterol is therefore considered the "good" cholesterol.

hollandaise sauce – Thick, rich sauce made of egg yolks, butter and lemon juice.

hypoglycemia - Abnormally low blood sugar.

incomplete protein - A protein source that is low in one or more of the essential amino acids.

iron - A mineral needed by the body to make the proteins hemoglobin and myoglobin. Hemoglobin is found in red blood cells, and myoglobin is found in muscles. They help carry and store oxygen in the body. Iron is also part of many other proteins and enzymes in the body.

kilocalorie (calorie) - A unit by which food energy is measured.

lacto-vegetarians - People who include milk or milk products but exclude meat, poultry, fish, seafood and eggs from their diets.

lacto-ovo-vegetarians- People who include milk or milk products and eggs but exclude meat, poultry, fish, and seafood from their diets.

lactose intolerance - A condition that results from inability to digest the milk sugar lactose; characterized by bloating, gas, abdominal discomfort and diarrhea.

low-density lipoprotein (LDL) – The lipoprotein that transports cholesterol from the liver to the tissues of the body. (Lipoproteins are the form in which lipids are transported in the blood.) LDL cholesterol is therefore considered the "bad" cholesterol.

macronutrient - A substance (such as protein, carbohydrate and fat) essential in large amounts for growth and health.

magnesium - A mineral that serves several important functions in the body: contraction and relaxation of muscles, function of certain enzymes in the body, production and transport of energy, production of protein.

metabolism - The sum of all the chemical reactions that occur in living cells.

micronutrient - An organic compound (such as vitamins and minerals) essential in minute amounts for growth and health.

monounsaturated fatty acid - A fatty acid that lacks two hydrogen atoms and has one double bond between carbons; found in liquid form at room temperature.

norepinephrine - A hormone secreted by certain nerve endings of the sympathetic nervous system and by the medulla (center) of the adrenal glands. Its primary function is to help maintain a constant blood pressure by stimulating certain blood vessels to constrict when the blood pressure falls below normal.

nutrient - A substance obtained from food and used in the body to provide energy and structural materials and to regulate growth, maintenance and repair of the body's tissues. The six classes of nutrients are carbohydrate, fat, protein, vitamins, minerals and water.

omega 3 fatty acid - A polyunsaturated fatty acid whose carbon chain has its first double-valence bond three carbons from the beginning; an essential fatty acid. DHA, EPA, and ALA are all omega 3 fatty acids.

organic food - Meat, poultry, eggs and dairy from animals that are given no antibiotics or growth hormones; plant foods produced without most conventional pesticides, fertilizers, synthetic ingredients or sewage sludge and not subject to bioengineering or ionizing radiation.

ovo-vegetarians - People who include eggs in their diet but exclude milk, milk products, meat, poultry, fish and seafood.

pan-fry - To cook over high heat in a small amount of fat.

percent (%) daily value (DV)- The percentage of the recommended daily allowance of a specific nutrient that a serving of food contains, based on a 2,000-calorie diet.

polyphenols - Any of a large class of organic compounds, of plant origin, having more than one phenol group. They tend to be colorful and to have antioxidant properties.

polyunsaturated fatty acid - A fatty acid that lacks four or more hydrogen atoms and has two or more double bonds between carbons; may be found in either a liquid or soft-solid form at room temperature.

poach - To cook in a hot liquid, being careful to retain the shape of the food (poached eggs or fish, for example).

potassium - An essential mineral that helps regulate heart function, blood pressure and nerve and muscle activity.

protein - A compound composed of carbon, hydrogen, oxygen and nitrogen atoms, arranged into amino acids linked in a chain; contains 4 calories per gram.

refined grains - Grains that have been milled, a process that removes the bran and germ. This is done to give grains a finer texture and improve their shelf life, but it also removes dietary fiber, iron and many B vitamins.

registered dietitian (RD) - A nutrition professional who has graduated from a university or college after completing a program of dietetics accredited by the American Dietetic Association, has served in an internship to practice the necessary skills, has passed the association's registration examination and maintains competency through continuing education.

roast - To cook uncovered in an oven.

saturated fat - Fat composed of triglycerides in which all or virtually all the fatty acids are saturated; usually solid at room temperature.

sauté - To brown or cook in a small amount of fat.

scallop - To bake food with a sauce or other liquid.

seitan - Wheat gluten.

selenium - A trace mineral that helps make special proteins, called antioxidant enzymes, which play a role in preventing cell damage.

simple carbohydrates - Carbohydrates that have one (single) or two (double) sugars. They are broken down quickly by the body to be used as energy. Simple carbohydrates are found naturally in foods such as fruits, milk, and milk products. They are also found in processed and refined sugars such as candy, table sugar, syrups and soft drinks.

serotonin - A neurotransmitter that regulates many functions, including mood, appetite and sensory perception.

sodium - A mineral and essential nutrient that helps to maintain blood volume, regulate the balance of water in the cells, and keep nerves functioning.

steam - To cook food in steam over boiling water in a closed container.

stir-fry - To fry thinly sliced food quickly in a small amount of oil, stirring with a tossing motion.

sugar alcohols - Naturally occurring sugar substitutes that have about half the calories of sugar. They get their name because they are carbohydrates that have a chemical structure similar to those of sugar and alcohol. Sugar alcohols are also referred to as polyols.

tempeh – A soy product made by a natural culturing and controlled fermentation process that binds soybeans into a cake form.

textured vegetable protein - A meat substitute made of defatted soy flour.

tofu - Soybean curd.

trans fatty acid - A fatty acid that has been produced by hydrogenating an unsaturated fatty acid (and so changing its shape); found in processed foods such as margarine, fried foods, commercially baked goods and partially hydrogenated vegetable oils.

triglyceride - A type of fat in the bloodstream and fat tissue.

tryptophan - An essential amino acid needed for normal growth; used to make niacin and serotonin.

tyrosine - An amino acid found in most proteins; a precursor of several hormones.

vegan - A person who excludes all animal-derived foods (including meat, poultry, fish, eggs and dairy products) from his diet.

vegetarian - A general term used to describe a person who excludes meat, poultry, fish or other animal-derived foods from his diet.

vitamin A - An antioxidant and fat-soluble vitamin with multiple functions in the body. It plays a role in vision, bone growth, reproduction, cell functions and the immune system.

vitamin C - An antioxidant required for the growth and repair of tissues in all parts of the body. It is necessary to form collagen, an important protein used to make skin, scar tissue, tendons, ligaments and blood vessels. Vitamin C is essential for the healing of wounds and for the repair and maintenance of cartilage, bones and teeth.

vitamin D - A fat-soluble vitamin that helps the body to absorb calcium and also has a role in the nerve, muscle and immune systems. Vitamin D can be obtained in three ways: through the skin, from your diet and from supplements. The body forms vitamin D naturally after exposure to sunlight.

vitamin E - An antioxidant and fat-soluble vitamin that plays a role in the immune system and metabolic processes.

wheat germ - The germ of the whole grain kernel.

white blood cells (leukocytes)- Blood cells that engulf and digest bacteria and fungi; an important part of the body's defense system.

whole-grain - Foods that contain all the essential parts (the bran, endosperm and germ) and naturally occurring nutrients of an entire grain seed.

zinc - An important trace mineral that the body's defensive (immune) system needs to properly work. It plays a role in cell division, cell growth, wound healing and the breakdown of carbohydrates. Zinc is also needed for the senses of smell and taste.

Resources

Food and exercise tracking (free):
 www.sparkpeople.com

Caloric and nutritional value of foods:
 www.calorieking.com

Calorie calculator:
 www.mayoclinic.com/health/calorie-calculator/nu00598

Food and nutrition information:
 www.eatright.org
 www.healthcastle.com
 www.mypyramid.gov
 www.nutrition.gov
 www.wholegrainscouncil.org

Recipe websites (quick and easy!):
 http://apps.nccd.cdc.gov/dnparecipe/recipesearch.aspx
 www.cookinglight.com/food/ quick-healthy/20-20-superfast-
  suppers-00400000038097/
 www.eatingwell.com/ http://www.foodnetwork.com/healthy-
  eating/index.html

Free coupons:
 www.coolsavings.com
 www.coupons.com
 www.couponsurfer.com

Health and medical:
 www.webmd.com
 www.mayoclinic.com
 www.healthfinder.gov
 http://symptoms.webmd.com

Promoting safety and wellness on campus (alcohol, drugs, sexual health, tobacco):
>   http://www.bacchusnetwork.org

Eating disorders:
>   National Eating Disorders Association:
>   www.nationaleatingdisorders.org
>   1-800-931-2237
>
>   Eating Disorders Anonymous:
>   www.eatingdisordersanonymous.org

Suicide Hotline: 1-800-784-2433

Grade-A Grocery List

Produce	-Apples -Apricots -Artichokes -Asparagus -Avocados -Beets -Baby carrots -Bananas -Bell Peppers -Berries -Broccoli -Brussels sprouts	-Cabbage -Cantaloupe -Cauliflower -Chard -Cherries -Cherry tomatoes -Celery -Collard greens -Cucumbers -Grapes -Grapefruit -Honeydew
Dairy, Soy, etc.	-1% or 2% Cottage Cheese -1% or skim milk -Soymilk -Almond milk -Rice milk	-1/3 Less Fat Cream Cheese -Block or shredded natural cheeses: Cheddar, Swiss, Mozzarella, String cheese
Frozen foods	-Fruit: Blueberries, Peaches, Strawberries (no added sugar) -Vegetables (no added salt) -Fudgesicles	-Skinny Cow frozen treats -Gorton's Grilled Fillets- Salmon or Tilapia -Kashi GoLean Frozen Waffles
Fresh meat, poultry, seafood	***Beef:*** -Round steak -95% lean ground beef -Chuck shoulder roast -Arm pot roast -Shoulder steak -Strip steak -Tenderloin steak -T-bone steak -Eye of round roast -Top round steak -Mock tender steak -Bottom round roast -Top sirloin steak	***Fish:*** -Crab -Haddock -Halibut -Mackerel -Salmon -Scallops -Shrimp -Tilapia -Trout -Tuna
Deli	-50% less sodium lunch meats (turkey, chicken or ham)	
Whole grain bread, pasta, rice, other grains	-Bob's Red Mill products -Brown Minute Rice -Brown Minute Rice (Ready to Serve) -Kashi 7 Grain Whole Pilaf -Mission Yellow Corn Tortillas	-Quick barley -Thomas' Hearty Grains 100% Whole Wheat Bagels -Thomas' Hearty Grains 100% Whole Wheat Bagels or Mini Bagels -Thomas' 100% Whole Wheat English Muffins

-Kale
-Kiwi
-Mango
-Mustard greens
-Nectarines
-Onions
-Oranges
-Papaya
-Peaches
-Pears
-Plums
-Pomegranates

-Potatoes (sweet/white)-Pumpkin
-Radishes
-Rutabagas
-Romaine Lettuce
-Spinach
-Squash
-Tangerines
-Turnip Greens
-Watermelon

-Butter
-Eggs
-Low-fat Greek Yogurt (Fage, Oiko's)

-Soy yogurt
-Margarine (trans fat free): Promise, Smart Balance

-MorningStar, Amy's Organic or Boca Veggie Burgers
-Natures Path Flax Plus Waffles

-Soybeans (Edamame)
-Tyson Ready Chicken-Grilled Chicken Breasts

Pork:
-Pork Tenderloin
-Pork boneless top loin chop
-Pork top loin roast
-Pork center loin chop
-Pork sirloin roast
-Pork rib chop

Poultry (skinless):
-Chicken breast
-Chicken leg
-Chicken thigh
-Turkey breast
-Turkey leg
-Turkey thigh

-Cheese by the slice: Cheddar, Swiss, Muenster, Colby

-Whole grain bread: 100% -Whole Wheat Country Hearth; 100% Whole Wheat Wonder Bread; Brownberry 100% Whole Wheat Bread
-Whole grain couscous
-Whole grain pasta (Barilla or Ronzi)
-Whole grain quinoa

-Whole grain tortillas
-Whole Wheat Pita (Aladdin's 100% Whole Wheat Pita)

Whole grain cereals	-Bran Flakes -Cascadia Cereals (any variety) -Cheerios -Fiber One Cereals -Grape Nut Flakes	-Frosted Mini Wheats -Grape Nuts -Kashi Cereals (any variety) -Kix
Whole grain granola bars and pasteries	-Cascadian Farms (any variety) -Fiber One Toaster Pastry -Kashi Granola Bars (any variety)	-Nature Valley Crunchy Granola Bars -Nutrigrain Bars
Whole Grain Crackers	-Kashi Heart to Heart Crackers -Triscuits Hint of Salt	-Wheat Thins -Miltons Whole Wheat Multigrain Crackers
Snacks	-Nuts: Walnuts, Pecans, Almonds, Peanuts -Pita Chips: Garden of Eatin' Whole Grain Pita Chips -Popcorn: Smart Balance Smart 'n Healthy Popcorn	-Pretzels: Snyder's of Hanover Whole Wheat & Oat Sticks or Honey Whole Wheat Sticks -Quaker Rice Cakes -Rice Works Gourmet Brown Rice Crisps
Cookies	-Archway Iced Lemonade -Archway Iced Molasses -Archway Iced Oatmeal	-Kashi Happy Trail Mix -Kashi Oatmeal Dark Chocolate
Canned & dry foods	-Applesauce cups -Beans: black, kidney, garbanzo, etc. -Canned fruit in juice or fruit cups in juice -Chicken of the Sea Salmon cups	-Dried fruit: Apricots, Pineapples, Plums, Figs, Raisins, Cranberry Raisins -Lentils -Lower Sodium Light Tuna
Beverages	-100% Apple Juice, Cranberry Juice, Grape Juice, Orange Juice (Ocean Spray, Tropicana) -Bottled water: Aquafina -Hint	-Naked Juice -Sobe 0 Calorie Lifewater
Condiments & oils	-Barbeque Sauce -Canola Oil -Ketchup	-Lower Sodium Soy Sauce -Mustard -Olive Oil
Other	-Agave Nectar -Bob's Red Mill Texturized Vegetable Protein -Calcium supplements (Viactiv or Caltrate)	-Chia Seeds -Flaxseed (milled): Hodgson Mill -Flintstone Vitamins

-Life -Quaker Oatmeal -Quaker Oatmeal Squares -Shredded Wheat	-Shredded Wheat Lightly Frosted -Total (any variety) -Wheaties
-PopTarts 20% Fiber -Quaker Simple Harvest	-Quaker True Delights
-Goldfish made with whole grains -Dr. Kracker	-Health Valley (Low Fat Whole Wheat) -Wasa Crackers Rye Crisp
-Shapers Whole Grain Chips: Black Bean & Salsa or Sea Salt -Smartfood Popcorn Clusters -Soy Crisps	-Sun Chips -Tortilla Chips: Garden of Eatin' Blue Chips; Snyder's Lightly Salted Tortilla Chips, Multigrain Lightly Salted Tortilla Chips or Eat Smart Naturals Multigrain Tortilla Chips; Corazones Whole Grain Tortilla Chips
-Kashi Oatmeal Raisin Flax -Newman's Own Cookies	-Snackwells Devil's Food Cookie Cake -Voortman Oatmeal Raisin (or any variety)
-Lower sodium soups: Campbell's Healthy Request Soup (50% less sodium) or Progresso 50% less sodium; V8 Soups (Tomato Herb; Sweet Red Pepper)	-Marinara sauce -Peanut butter: Smucker's Natural -Planters Lightly Salted Peanuts -Tyson or Swanson white canned chicken
-V8 Fusion	
-Olive Oil Mayonnaise -Olives -Pickles	-Salad Dressing: Balsamic Vinaigrette, Italian -Salsa
-Hershey's Bliss Dark Chocolate -Hummus (Sabra, Tribe, Athenos) -True Lemon	-Wheat germ

Brain-Building Foods

Brain-Building Carbs:
-Whole-grain cereals, crackers, bread, pasta, oats, brown rice, etc. -Fruit (fresh or frozen rather than juice) -Legumes: dried beans, peas and lentils -Milk and yogurt -Vegetables

Brain-Building Fats:	
Monounsaturated Fats: Avocados Canola oil Nuts Olive oil Olives Peanut oil Seeds Sunflower oil	**Polyunsaturated Fats:** Corn oil Most nuts and seeds Safflower oil

Omega 3 fatty acids:

DHA/EPA-rich:	ALA-rich:
Herring	Canola oil
Mackerel	Flaxseed oil
Salmon	Soybean oil
Sardines	Chia seeds
Trout	Flaxseed
Tuna	Pumpkin seeds
	Soybeans
	Tofu
	Walnuts
	Omega 3 eggs

Brain-Building Vitamins:		
	Food Sources	
Vitamin B1—Thiamin	Dairy products Enriched grains Fish Fruits Lean meats Legumes	Nuts and seeds Soybeans Vegetables Wheat germ Whole grains
Vitamin B2—Riboflavin	Cottage cheese Enriched grains Leafy greens Meat	Milk Whole grains Yogurt
Vitamin B3—Niacin	Eggs Enriched grains Fish Lean meats Legumes	Milk Nuts Poultry Whole grains

Brain-Building Vitamins: Food Sources		
Vitamin B5—Pantothenic acid	Broccoli and other vegetables in the cabbage family Eggs Fish	Lean beef Legumes Milk and milk products Poultry Whole-grain cereals
Vitamin B6—Pyridoxine	Fish and shellfish Fruits Leafy greens Legumes	Meats Poultry Whole grains
Vitamin B7—Biotin	Broccoli and other vegetables in the cabbage family Eggs Fish	Lean beef Legumes Milk and milk products Whole-grain cereals
Vitamin B9—Folate/Folic Acid	Citrus fruits Leafy greens Legumes	Seeds Whole grains
Vitamin B12—Cobalamin	Animal products (meat, fish, poultry, shellfish, milk, cheese, eggs, yogurt)	Fortified grains
Choline	Egg yolk Liver Soybeans	Wheat germ Whole-wheat products

Immune-Boosting Foods

Vitamin A-Rich Foods *Antioxidant*	Apricots Asparagus Beet greens Broccoli Cantaloupe Carrots Cherries Corn	Green Peppers Kale Mangoes Nectarines Peaches Pink grapefruit Pumpkin Romaine Lettuce	Spinach Squash Sweet potatoes Tangerines Tomatoes Turnip/collard greens Watermelon
Vitamin C-Rich Foods *Antioxidant*	Berries Broccoli Brussels sprouts Cabbage Cantaloupe Cauliflower Grapefruit	Honeydew Kale Kiwi Mangoes Mustard greens Nectarines Oranges	Papaya Peppers Rutabagas Snow peas Strawberries Sweet potatoes Tomatoes
Vitamin B6—Pyridoxine	Fish & shellfish Fruits Leafy greens	Legumes Meats	Poultry Whole grains
Vitamin B9— Folate/Folic Acid	Citrus fruits Leafy greens	Legumes Seeds	Whole grains
Vitamin E-Rich Foods *Antioxidant*	Broccoli Carrots Chard Fortified cereals Mangoes	Margarine Mustard greens Nuts Papaya Pumpkin	Red peppers Spinach Sunflower seeds Turnip greens Vegetable oils Wheat germ
Copper	Beans Fish	Nuts and seeds Organ meats (kidneys, liver)	Oysters and other shellfish Whole grains
Iron	Red meat Egg yolk Dark leafy greens (spinach, collards)	Dried fruit (prunes, raisins) Iron-enriched cereals and grains Shellfish	Poultry Beans, lentils, soybeans Liver
Zinc	Beans Beef (lean) Crab Eggs	Fish Fortified cereals Milk Nuts	Oysters Poultry Tofu Wheat germ Yogurt

Omega 3 Fatty Acid-Rich Foods	DHA/EPA-rich: Herring Mackerel Salmon Sardines Trout Tuna		ALA-rich: Canola oil Flaxseed oil Soybean oil Chia Seeds Flaxseed Omega 3 eggs Pumpkin seeds Soybeans Tofu Walnuts
Selenium-Rich Foods *Antioxidant*	Beans/legumes Beef Garlic Shrimp Brazil nuts Tuna	Brown rice Lobster Vegetables Chicken Whole grains	Cottage cheese Nuts/seeds Egg yolk Red snapper Poultry
Yogurt	Plain yogurt	Greek yogurt	Flavored yogurt
	Offers healthy bacteria to stimulate white blood cells		

Stress-Busting Foods

Food:	How does it help your stress?	Sources of:	
B-vitamin-rich foods	✓ It maintains nerve and brain cells and converts the food you eat into energy you can use. ✓ You need it to make serotonin	Broccoli Cheese Cottage cheese Eggs Enriched grains Fish Fruits Leafy greens Lean meats	Legumes Milk Nuts Poultry Seeds Shellfish Soybeans Whole grains Yogurt
Choline-rich foods	✓ Helps with memory ✓ Reduces inflammation	Egg yolk Liver Soybeans	Wheat germ Whole-wheat products
Water	✓ You need it to convert food into energy	Bottled water Tap water	Flavored water (calorie-free)

Food:	How does it help your stress?	Sources of:		
Omega 3 fatty acid-rich foods	✓ Higher blood levels of omega 3 fatty acids have been linked to better mood	**DHA/EPA-rich:** Herring Mackerel Salmon Sardines Trout Tuna	**ALA-rich:** Canola oil Flaxseed oil Soybean oil Chia seeds Flaxseed Omega 3 eggs	Pumpkin seeds Soybeans Tofu Walnuts
Whole grains	✓ Boosts serotonin, the "feel-good" brain chemical	Barley Brown rice Oatmeal Popcorn Quinoa	WG cereals WG crackers WG bread WG pasta	
Vitamin C-rich foods	✓ Contain antioxidants, which fight free radicals that are released when you're stressed	Berries Broccoli Brussels sprouts Cabbage Cantaloupe Cauliflower Grapefruit Honeydew Kale Kiwi	Mangoes Mustard greens Nectarines Oranges Papaya Peppers Rutabagas Snow peas Strawberries Sweet potatoes Tomatoes	
Vitamin E-rich foods	✓ Contain antioxidants, which fight free radicals that are released when you're stressed	Broccoli Carrots Chard Fortified cereals Mangoes Margarine Mustard greens Nuts	Papaya Pumpkin Red peppers Spinach Turnip greens Sunflower seeds Vegetable oils Wheat germ	
Magnesium	✓ Relaxes muscles and nerves ✓ Stress depletes this mineral	Beans Halibut Nuts Seeds	Soybeans Spinach Wheat germ Whole grains	
Selenium	✓ Repairs oxidative damage caused by stress	Beans/legumes Beef Garlic Shrimp Brazil nuts Tuna Brown rice Lobster	Vegetables Chicken Whole grains Cottage cheese Nuts/seeds Egg yolk Red snapper Poultry	

Just Plain Good-for-You Foods (Antioxidant-Rich)

Apples with skin	Cabbage	Guava	Potatoes with skin
Apricots (dried)	Cherries	Kiwi	(sweet and white)
Artichokes	Currants	Mangoes	Prunes/plums
Asparagus	Dark chocolate	Nuts	Radishes
Avocados	Figs	Oats	Raisins
Beans and legumes	Garlic	Onions	Red cabbage
Beets	Grapefruit	Oranges	Red wine
Bell peppers	Grapes	Peaches	Spices
Berries	Green leafy lettuce	Pears	Spinach
Broccoli	Green tea	Pomegranates	

Common Portion Equivalents

Common portion equivalent	Serving size	Equals 1 portion of
Truffle	1 tablespoon	Peanut butter
Baseball	1 cup	-Fruit or vegetables -Cereal (flakes or rounds)
Golf ball	2 tablespoons	Hummus
Computer mouse	1 each	Size of a medium potato
Deck of cards or an iPhone	3 oz.	Beef or chicken
Checkbook	3 oz.	Fish
Stamp	1 teaspoon	Oil
Tennis ball	½ cup	-Beans or potatoes -Hot cereal -Cooked pasta or rice -Dried fruit
6 stacked dice	1½ oz.	Cheese
Egg	¼ cup	-Beans (1 oz. meat) -Granola
CD	1 each	Pancake or waffle
Yo-yo	1 oz.	Dinner roll
Hockey puck	1 oz.	Half a medium bagel

Food Journal

Hunger or fullness level before I ate (1-10)	What did I eat? What did I drink?

Hunger or fullness level when I stopped eating (1-10)	How am I feeling? Sad, happy, depressed, angry, lonely, stressed, etc.	If I am feeding my "head hunger," how can I cope next time?

Food Journal

Hunger or fullness level before I ate (1-10)	What did I eat? What did I drink?

Hunger or fullness level when I stopped eating (1-10)	How am I feeling? Sad, happy, depressed, angry, lonely, stressed, etc.	If I am feeding my "head hunger," how can I cope next time?

Food-Tracking Sheet

Meal	Menu	Meat/ Beans (oz.)	Grains (oz.)	Milk (cups)
Breakfast				
Snack				
Lunch				
Snack				
Dinner				
Snack				
Totals:				

Fruit (cups)	Vegetables (cups)	Healthy Fat (tsp)	Omega 3's ♥	Water (oz.)	Extras (Calories)

Food-Tracking Sheet

Meal	Menu	Meat/ Beans (oz.)	Grains (oz.)	Milk (cups)
Breakfast				
Snack				
Lunch				
Snack				
Dinner				
Snack				
Totals:				

Fruit (cups)	Vegetables (cups)	Healthy Fat (tsp)	Omega 3's ♥	Water (oz.)	Extras (Calories)

Power Habit™ Tracking Chart

Day	Power Habit(s)™ I will focus on	Number of exercise minutes

Power Habit™ Tracking Chart

Day	Power Habit(s)™ I will focus on	Number of exercise minutes

Power Habit™ Tracking Chart

Day	Power Habit(s)™ I will focus on	Number of exercise minutes

Power Habit™ Tracking Chart

Day	Power Habit(s)™ I will focus on	Number of exercise minutes

Power Habit™ Tracking Chart

Day	Power Habit(s)™ I will focus on	Number of exercise minutes

Power Habit™ Tracking Chart

Day	Power Habit(s)™ I will focus on	Number of exercise minutes

Power Habits™

READ IT POWER HABITS™!

✓ Read the food labels of every food you consider eating today.

✓ Choose those with a 20% or higher DV for fiber, calcium, iron, vitamin A and/or vitamin C.

✓ Choose those with less than a 20% DV for total fat, saturated fat, cholesterol and/or sodium.

✓ For fun, calculate the percentage of carbohydrate, protein, fat and saturated fat in a couple of food products to see how they match up with the recommendations.

✓ Opt for foods labeled with "Reduced," "Good source of," "High in" and "High fiber".

✓ Write your own Read It Power Habit™: _____

SMART-FAT POWER HABITS™!

✓ Replace fried chicken and other breaded and fried foods with grilled or baked ones. Don't forget to remove the skin!

✓ Choose grilled or stir-fried veggies or baked potatoes over french fries.

✓ Read food labels for trans fats! Eliminate foods with partially hydrogenated vegetable oils.

✓ Choose healthier mono and polyunsaturated fats. Grab a small handful of peanuts instead of potato chips or snack mix.

✓ Eat fish twice a week. If you haven't learned to love fish yet, include walnuts or ground flaxseed in your meals and snacks. Mix walnuts into your oatmeal, and sprinkle flaxseed on your salad or mix it into your yogurt.

✓ Limit high-fat dairy products. To save on saturated fat, go for skim or 1% milk instead of 2% or whole. If you eat cheese, keep the portions small (1½ ounces of hard cheese is the size of six stacked dice).

✓ Write your own Smart-Fat Power Habit™: _____

SALT SHAKIN' POWER HABITS™!

✓ Shelve the salt shaker. Use unsalted spices and herbs to flavor your foods.

✓ Choose lower-sodium soups and snacks.

✓ Eat your fruits and veggies! They're loaded with potassium, which helps blunt sodium's effects on your blood pressure.

✓ Eat fresh or frozen vegetables instead of canned.

✓ If you eat canned foods like beans, vegetables or olives, rinse them under cold water to remove some of the sodium.

✓ Read food labels for sodium!

✓ Eat fewer processed meats like deli meats, hot dogs and sausage and choose more fresh meats like chicken and fish.

✓ Write your own Salt Shakin' Power Habit™: _____

_____

WHOLE GRAIN POWER HABITS™!

✓ Go whole grain! When choosing bread, cereal or pasta, be sure the first word on the list of ingredients is "whole".

✓ Visit the Whole Grains Council and look for your favorite cereal or granola bar. www.wholegrainscouncil.org

✓ Choose brown rice instead of white rice.

✓ Eat a bowl of oatmeal for breakfast.

✓ Snack on whole grain chips like SunChips instead of potato chips.

✓ Order your sandwich or wrap on whole grain bread or in a whole grain tortilla.

✓ Toss a whole grain cereal bar like Kashi Honey Almond & Flax into your bag for a quick snack between classes.

✓ Write your own Whole Grain Power Habit™: _____

_____

LEAN PROTEIN POWER HABITS™!

✓ Opt for grilled, baked, poached, broiled or roasted meats, and go easy on the sauces.

✓ Go fish for a powerful brain! Try it just one time a week for starters.

✓ Combine your carbohydrates with lean protein for maximum energy and focus.

✓ Choose more fresh-meat sandwiches and fewer deli meats.

✓ Snacks need protein, too. Instead of a handful of baby carrots, how about adding a hard-boiled egg or a handful of nuts or seeds on the side?

✓ Try soybeans on your salad or a soy burger for lunch.

✓ Write your own Lean Protein Power Habit™: _____

BONE-BANKING POWER HABITS™!

✓ If you don't like plain milk, blend 1% or skim milk with fruit and yogurt for a calcium-loaded smoothie.

✓ Eat string cheese for your afternoon snack.

✓ For a great midmorning snack, stir a small handful of peanuts and low-fat granola into a container of your favorite low-fat yogurt.

✓ Make it skinny! Order your latte or mocha with skim milk instead of 2% or whole milk.

✓ Use milk instead of water when making pancakes, oatmeal or Cream of Wheat.

✓ Write you our own Bone-Banking Power Habit™: _____

FRUIT TOOTH POWER HABITS™!

✓ Stock your kitchen or dorm room with fresh fruit for when your sweet tooth attacks. Apples, bananas, pears, oranges and grapes are all very portable.

✓ If you can't get fresh fruit, fill your freezer with frozen fruit like strawberries, blueberries and peaches. If you don't have much freezer space, try unsweetened applesauce and dried fruit.

✓ For a snack, grab a cluster of grapes instead of a handful of M&M's.

✓ Top your morning bowl of oatmeal with sliced strawberries or a handful of raisins.

✓ When fruit just won't cut the craving and you must have candy, try a square of dark chocolate.

✓ Write your own Fruit Tooth Power Habit™: _____

_____

VEG OUT POWER HABITS™!

✓ When you dine out, order a side of vegetables rather than a side of french fries.

✓ Make it a habit to fill a 3-cup food container with raw vegetables every day and snack on them when you get hungry. Baby carrots, sliced cucumbers, red pepper strips and cherry tomatoes all work great. If you need dip, try hummus.

✓ Most campus dining halls have a salad bar. Either have a salad with your meal or make it the main course by adding black beans and grilled chicken on top.

✓ When you make or order a smoothie, toss a handful of baby carrots or spinach into the blender along with skim milk and fruit. Not only does it make for a thicker consistency, but it also keeps you full for longer.

✓ Low-sodium V8 juice is a great snack you can carry in your bag. It comes in convenient 4-ounce cans and counts as a half-cup of vegetables.

✓ Write your own Veg Out Power Habit™: _____

_____

H$_2$O POWER HABITS™!

✓ Replace that 12-ounce can of soda with 12 ounces of water.

✓ Make it a habit to carry a water bottle with you to class and sip on it throughout the day.

✓ If you like your water with a little flavor, drop in a cucumber slice or squeeze a few drops of lemon, lime or orange juice into it. True Lemon makes small packets of crystallized lemon, lime and orange to mix into your water for flavor without the calories or artificial sweeteners.

✓ If you choose a fruit drink or other sugary beverage, dilute it with water.

✓ Drink 8 ounces of water between each of your meals.

✓ Drink 8 ounces of water with each of your meals.

✓ Write your own H$_2$O Power Habit™: _____

GO WITH YOUR GUT POWER HABITS™!

✓ Redefine your gas tank. Use the 1-5 scale instead of 1-10.

✓ Be mindful when you eat today. Assign a number to your hunger and fullness and get to know your level "4."

✓ Slow down! Savor each bite. Remember, the faster you eat, the more you eat.

✓ Drink 8 to 16 ounces of water before a meal and before you reach for a snack. You may actually be thirsty or dehydrated, not hungry.

✓ During meals, pick a place to eat, like your kitchen table, a dining-hall table or at your desk, and do only that—eat!

✓ Mind your portions. Match your portion sizes with common objects (see chart) to be sure you aren't overeating.

✓ If you find yourself eating when you aren't hungry, find out why and develop a new coping skill. Put the skill to use every time you reach for food to feed your head hunger.

✓ Write your own Go With Your Gut Power Habit™: _____

BUTT-MOVIN' POWER HABITS™!

✓ Schedule exercise time on your calendar like you do your classes and commit.

✓ Take the stairs instead of the elevator at every opportunity. If you live on the fourth floor of your residence hall or apartment, think of how many calories you'll burn if you take the stairs every day. Remember, the 30-minutes-a-day exercise recommendation can be spread out. Five minutes here and there all count toward the total!

✓ Find an exercise buddy and work out with him or her at scheduled times each week. You'll be much less likely to skip when your friend is counting on you.

✓ Lace up your tennis shoes and walk! Walking to class counts if you're doing it briskly enough to raise your heart rate.

✓ Take advantage of your campus recreation center. Whether you prefer swimming, group exercise classes, the treadmill or the elliptical machine, your campus fitness center is one of the true gems at your university. If you don't know how to work a piece of exercise equipment, ask a fitness-center staff person.

✓ Write your own Butt-Movin' Power Habit™: _____

BRAIN-BUILDING POWER HABITS™!

✓ Eat only brain-building carbohydrates today. If you can't stop yourself from indulging in a brain-draining carb like soda or a cookie, be sure to eat or drink it after your meal to weaken the serotonin effect.

✓ Don't skip meals, especially breakfast. If you're in a hurry and have to eat on the go, grab a Kashi Honey Almond Flax bar and wash it down with 8 ounces of skim milk (226 calories, 54% carbohydrate, 26% protein, 20% fat).

✓ To rev up your brain in the morning, eat a light breakfast with some lean protein and brain-building carbohydrates (example: a three-egg-white omelet with 1 ounce of Cheddar cheese, a half-cup of black beans and a small banana).

✓ To get your B-vitamins, be sure to eat a few servings of whole grains today.

✓ Whether it's for breakfast or as a snack, find a way to eat an egg today to boost your choline (and your memory, too).

✓ Keep it light! Large meals equal heavy eyes.

✓ Sweep up the free radicals in your body with antioxidant-rich foods. Pick three from the list to include in your diet today.

✓ Write your own Brain-Building Power Habit™: _____

IMMUNE-BOOSTING POWER HABITS™!

✓ Eat at least 1½ cups of fruit and 2 cups of vegetables every day.

✓ Eat a 6-ounce container of yogurt as a snack.

✓ Sprinkle some crushed walnuts or 1 tablespoon of milled flaxseeds on your oatmeal.

✓ Choose salmon or tuna instead of beef or chicken.

✓ Schedule exercise into your day and make it a priority. Start by committing to three days a week and build from there.

✓ Get at least seven hours of sleep each night.

✓ Watch the added sugars in your diet, especially soda! Choose water instead.

✓ Write your own Immune-Boosting Power Habit™: _____

STRESS-BUSTING POWER HABITS™!

✓ Make a list of all the ways you dance around your stress instead of dancing with it. Formulate a plan to tackle each one. What can you do instead?

✓ Instead of stuffing your face, do something positive (like calling a positive friend) to cope with your stress.

✓ Have healthy, stress-busting foods on hand in your dorm or apartment. Choose a nutritious and balanced snack if you must eat in response to stress.

✓ Get at least seven hours of sleep every night.

✓ Make time for exercise, especially if you expect to have an extra-stressful day.

✓ Realize that there are only 24 hours in the day. Don't put so much on your plate if you know there's no way you'll get it all done. Prioritize!

✓ Write your own Stress-Busting Power Habit™: _____

LEAN DINING-HALL POWER HABITS™!

✓ Pass on the muffin for breakfast and fill up on a whole-grain English muffin or bagel with a smear of peanut butter instead.

✓ Fill your lunch or dinner plate with half veggies, a quarter lean meat, beans or soy and a quarter whole grain or starchy vegetable.

✓ Opt for whole-grain bread and pasta or brown rice instead of regular. To ease yourself into it, try asking for half whole-grain pasta or brown rice and the other half regular.

✓ Choose marinara or light garlic olive oil sauce instead of alfredo or other cream sauces.

✓ Choose broth-based soups over creamy soups for lunch and dinner.

✓ Slash 200 calories by drinking water with your meals instead of soda or fruit punch.

✓ Write your own Lean Dining Hall Power Habit™: _____

PLAN YOUR PLATE POWER HABITS™!

✓ Visit the Web site www.mayoclinic.com/health/calorie-calculator/nu00598 to determine how many calories your body requires to stay at its current weight.

✓ Eat breakfast every day, and be sure to include an ounce of protein.

✓ Choose the "better" or "best" option at lunch or dinner today.

✓ Get a feel for what a portion is supposed to look like by comparing all the foods you eat today with the standard portion sizes listed in the Food Lists. Are they larger, smaller or about the right size?

✓ Use the Power Meal Plates™ as a guide to plan one of your meals today.

✓ Fill half your lunch and dinner plates with colorful vegetables like broccoli.

✓ Eat healthy and energizing snacks between meals to keep your energy up.

✓ Write your own Plan Your Plate Power Habit™: _____

GRADE-A SHOPPING POWER HABITS™!

✓ Always shop from a list! Use the Grade-A Grocery List in the appendix and highlight the foods you plan to buy.

✓ Load your cart with healthy proteins and carbohydrates so that you'll always have good food available for a quick snack.

✓ Limit junk food to one purchase.

✓ Since you're probably sharing a refrigerator, limit your perishable food items to milk, yogurt, cheese, fresh fruits and vegetables, veggie burgers and frozen vegetables.

✓ Put a stop to impulse purchases—eat something before you shop.

✓ Kashi products are your best friends. Look for Kashi granola bars, cereal, cookies and crackers.

✓ Read the food label before putting it in your cart.

✓ Write your own Grade-A Shopping Power Habit™: _____

HEALTHY FAST FOOD POWER HABITS™!

✓ Since restaurant portions are often huge, split the meal with a friend and save on calories and money or ask for a doggie bag!

✓ Opt for grilled, baked, stir-fried, broiled, roasted or steamed instead of fried, deep-fried, crispy, battered, creamy or sautéed.

✓ Ask for non-creamy dressing for your salad (on the side), and use only half.

✓ Just say no to supersized meals.

✓ Choose fish and skinless poultry over beef and pork.

✓ Order your favorite coffee drink with skim or 1% milk.

✓ Ask for whole-wheat bread or pasta and brown rice instead of white.

✓ Skip the heavy sauces and gravies.

✓ Ask for a side of veggies instead of french fries.

✓ Treat beverages just like food and don't overdrink. Choose water or skim milk. If you must have a soda, limit it to one and ask for lots of ice.

✓ Write your own Healthy Fast Food Power Habit™: _____

VEGETARIAN POWER HABITS™!

✓ If you're a vegan, be sure to get plenty of calcium. Three cups (8 ounces) of low-fat calcium-fortified soy, rice or almond milk each day will do the trick.

✓ Take a daily multivitamin and calcium supplement with added vitamin D, especially if you think you aren't regularly eating vegetarian sources of calcium, iron, vitamin D, vitamin B-12 and zinc.

✓ Don't shy away from certain menu items like grilled chicken salad or spaghetti and meatballs just because they have meat in them. Ask for the dish anyway, but without the meat. If the restaurant serves beans, lentils or veggie burgers, request that your meal be topped with one of those instead.

✓ Eat a bowl of fortified cereal like Total every day.

✓ To stay satisfied, eat a serving of protein such as tofu, beans or an egg at each meal.

✓ Combine plant sources of iron with vitamin C for best absorption. For example: black beans and rice with diced tomatoes.

✓ Be sure to eat one to two servings of walnuts, soybeans and other vegetarian sources of omega 3 fatty acids every day.

✓ Write your own Vegetarian Power Habit™: _____

_____

References

Secret 1

US Food and Drug Administration. **How to understand and use the nutrition facts label.** U.S. Food and Drug Administration website http://www.fda.gov/food/labelingnutrition/consumerinformation/ucm078889. htm November 2004; Accessed June 11, 2010

Kratz M. **Dietary cholesterol, atherosclerosis and coronary heart disease.** *Handb Exp Pharmacol* 2005:195-213

RD 411. **Muscle Building: Does Protein Play a Role?** RD 411 website http://www.rd411.com/index.php?option=com_content&view=article &id=172:muscle-building:-does-protein-play-a-role?&catid=78:sports-nutrition&Itemid=357 November 2008; Accessed June 10, 2010

Heaney RP. **Role of Dietary Sodium in Osteoporosis.** *Journal of the American College of Nutrition* 2006: 271S-276S

Secret 2

American Heart Association. American Heart Association website http://www.heart.org/HEARTORG/

United States Department of Agriculture. USDA website http://www.mypyramid.gov/

Kris-Etherton PM, Hill AM. **n-3 fatty acids: Food or supplements?** *J Am Diet Assoc.* 2008; 1125-1130

Grandgirard A, Bourre JM, Julliard F, Homayoun P, Dumont O. **Incorporation of Trans Long-Chain n-3 Polyunsaturated Fatty Acids in Rat Brain Structures and Retina.** *Lipids,* 1994; 251-58

Secret 3

National Institutes of Health. **Too much salt.** NIH Medline Plus website http://www.nlm.nih.gov/medlineplus/magazine/issues/sprsum10/articles/ sprsum10pg14.html Spring/Summer 2010; Accessed July 30, 2010

American Heart Association. American Heart Association website http://www.heart.org/HEARTORG/

Secret 4

Whole Grains Council. Whole Grains Council website http://www.wholegrainscouncil.org/

United States Department of Agriculture. USDA website
http://www.mypyramid.gov/

Cansev M, Wurtman RJ. **Aromatic Amino Acids in the Brain**. 2007,
Handbook of Neurochemistry and Molecular Neurobiology. 2007; 59-97

Web MD. *Serotonin: 9 Questions and Answers* Web MD website
http://www.webmd.com/depression/recognizing-depression-symptoms/serotonin
October 2010; Accessed November 1, 2010

Secret 5

United States Department of Agriculture. USDA website
http://www.mypyramid.gov/

American Heart Association. American Heart Association website
http://www.heart.org/HEARTORG/

Fernstrom JD. **Dietary Amino Acids and Brain Function**. *J Am Diet Assoc.*
1994; 71-77.

Fernstrom JD, Fernstrom M. **Tyrosine, phenylalanine, and catecholamine
synthesis and function in the brain**. J. Nutr. 2007: 1539S-1547S

Committee on Military Nutrition Research. **Food Components to Enhance
Performance** The National Academies Press website
http://www.nap.edu/openbook.php?record_id=4563&page=279
http://www.nap.edu/openbook.php?record_id=4563&page=337
1994; Accessed September 15, 2010

Harvard School of Public Health. *Red and Processed Meat Consumption
and Risk of Incident Coronary Heart Disease, Stroke, and Diabetes Mellitus.
A Systematic Review and Meta-Analysis* Circulation website http://circ.
ahajournals.org/cgi/content/abstract/CIRCULATIONAHA.109.924977v1
May 2010; Accessed March 4, 2011

Secret 6

Office of Dietary Supplements National Institutes of Health. **Dietary
supplement fact sheet: Vitamin D**. Office of Dietary Supplements website
http://ods.od.nih.gov/factsheets/vitamind/ February 2011;
Accessed March 4, 2011

Office of Dietary Supplements National Institutes of Health. **Dietary
supplement fact sheet: Calcium**. Office of Dietary Supplements website
http://ods.od.nih.gov/factsheets/Calcium-QuickFacts/ March 2011 and http://
ods.od.nih.gov/factsheets/calcium/ January 2011; Accessed both April 1, 2011

American Dietetic Association. **Position of the American Dietetic Association and Dietitians of Canada: Nutrition and Women's Health** *J Am Diet Assoc.* 2004; 984-1001

United States Department of Agriculture. USDA website http://www.mypyramid.gov/

Secret 7

United States Department of Agriculture. USDA website http://www.mypyramid.gov/

Yang Q. **Gain Weight By "Going Diet?" Artificial Sweeteners and the Neurobiology of Sugar Cravings.** *Yale J Biol Med.* 2010; 101-108

Mayo Clinic. **Artificial sweeteners: Understanding these and other sugar substitutes.** Mayo Clinic website http://www.mayoclinic.com/health/artificial-sweeteners/MY00073 October 2010; Accessed March 19, 2011

Gearhardt AN, Corbin WR, Brownell KD. **Preliminary validation of the Yale Food Addiction Scale.** *Appetite.* 2009; 430-436

Secret 8

Poon HF, Calabrese V, Scapagnini G, Butterfield DA. **Free Radicals and Brain Aging.** *Clin Geriatr Med.* 2004; 329-59

Emerit I. **Free Radicals and Aging of the Skin.** *EXS.* 1992; 328-341

Secret 9

Kleiner SM. **Water: An essential but overlooked nutrient.** *J Am Diet Assoc.* 1999; 200-206

Merck. **Dehydration.** The Merck Manuels Online Medical Library http://www.merckmanuals.com/home/sec12/ch158/ch158b.html August 2008; Accessed December 21, 2010

Position of the American Dietetic Association, Dietitians of Canada, and the American College of Sports Medicine: Nutrition and Athletic Performance. *J Am Diet Assoc.* 2009; 509-527

Secret 11

Keim NL, Blanton CA, Kretsch MJ. **America's obesity epidemic: Measuring physical activity to promote an active lifestyle.** *J Am Diet Assoc.* 2004; 1398-1409

Calabrese LH. **Exercise, immunity and infection.** *Journal of the American Osteopathic Association.* 1996; 166-176

Cotman CW, Berchtold NC, Christie L. **Exercise Builds Brain Health: Key Roles of Growth Factor Cascades and Inflammation.** *Trends in Neurosciences.* 2007; 464-472

Secret 12

National Institute on Alcohol Abuse and Alcoholism. **Influence of Alcohol and Gender on Immune Response.** NIAAA website http://pubs.niaaa.nih.gov/publications/arh26-4/257-263.htm June 2003; Accessed December 9, 2010

National Institute on Alcohol Abuse and Alcoholism. **Alcohol Alert.** NIAAA website http://pubs.niaaa.nih.gov/publications/aa22.htm October 1993; Accessed December 9, 2010

Reissig CJ, Strain EC, Griffiths RR. **Caffeinated Energy Drinks—A Growing Problem.** *Drug Alcohol Depend.* 2009; 1-10

Secret 13

Committee on Military Nutrition Research. **Food Components to Enhance Performance** The National Academies Press website http://www.nap.edu/openbook.php?record_id=4563&page=279 http://www.nap.edu/openbook.php?record_id=4563&page=388 1994; Accessed September 15, 2010

The Free Library by Farlex. **Food and Mood.** The Free Library website http://www.thefreelibrary.com/Food+%26+mood.-a012520128 1992; Accessed February 22, 2011

Wilson MMG, Morley JE. **Impaired Cognitive Function and Mental Performance in Mild Dehydration.** *European Journal of Clinical Nutrition.* 2003; S24-S29

Kempton MJ, Ettinger U, Foster R, Williams SC, Calvert GA, Hampshire A, Zelaya FO, O'Gorman RL, McMorris T, Owen AM, Smith MS. **Dehydration affects brain structure and function in healthy adolescents.** *Hum Brain Mapp.* 2011; 71-79

Fernstrom JD, Fernstrom M. **Tyrosine, phenylalanine, and catecholamine synthesis and function in the brain.** J. Nutr. 2007: 1539S-1547S

Secret 14

Web MD. **10 Immune System Boosters and Busters.** Web MD website http://www.webmd.com/cold-and-flu/10-immune-system-busters-boosters November 2009; Accessed January 9, 2011

Today's Dietitian. **Cortisol—Its Role in Stress, Inflammation, and Indications for Diet Therapy.** Today's Dietitian website http://www.todaysdietitian.com/newarchives/111609p38.shtml November 2009; Accessed February 26, 2011

Secret 17

United States Department of Agriculture. USDA website http://www.mypyramid.gov/

Secret 19

www.arbys.com
www.bk.com
www.chipotle.com
www.kfc.com
www.longjohnsilvers.com
www.mcdonalds.com
www.papajohns.com
www.paneranutrition.com
www.starbucks.com
www.subway.com
www.tacobell.com
www.wendys.com
www.pandaexpress.com
www.outback.com
www.olivegarden.com

Secret 20

United States Department of Agriculture. USDA website http://www.mypyramid.gov/

Vegetarian Resource Group. VRG website www.vrg.org

Secret 21

National Eating Disorders Association. NEDA website www.nationaleatingdisorders.org

Eating Disorders Anonymous. Eating Disorders Anonymous website www.eatingdisordersanonymous.org

INDEX

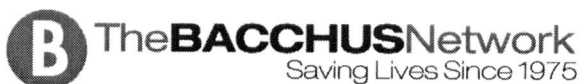

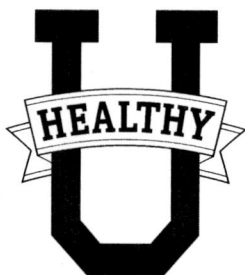

To order additional copies go to:
www.healthyUbook.com